# The Long Arc of Training

*The Long Arc of Training* follows six medical trainees over twelve years, capturing the peaks, valleys, and plateaus in their transformative journey from classrooms to independent clinical practice. Using repeated interviews across that span, the book captures the deeply human side of medical training. Its not just what these six aspiring doctors learn, but how they become who they are.

Unlike memoirs written in hindsight or short-term studies, this book presents longitudinal narratives that unfold gradually. Readers witness how the emotional responses, sense of self, personal well-being, and career plans of doctors-in-the making transform alongside growing medical knowledge and clinical skills.

This book is for anyone curious about the process of becoming a doctor – aspiring medical students, current trainees, practicing physicians, educators, and readers drawn to stories of growth and transformation. With a focus on authentic storytelling, *The Long Arc of Training* challenges common assumptions about medical education and invites reflection on how to best support those in training. It provides a fresh, human-centered perspective on a process often viewed in purely academic terms.

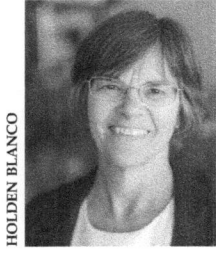

DORENE F. BALMER is professor of pediatrics at the Perelman School of Medicine at the University of Pennsylvania, and co-director of research, CHOP Education Collaboratory at the Children's Hospital of Philadelphia.

# Praise for *The Long Arc of Training*

"Balmer's *The Long Arc of Training* is a transformational, all-too-rare look at the gradual, often invisible process of becoming a doctor, and the necessity of conducting sustained, longitudinal work in adequately capturing that metamorphosis. Her fifteen-year journey of discovery is both a North Star and role model for future researchers."
    Frederic W. Hafferty, Senior Fellow, Center for Professionalism and the Future of Medicine, Accreditation Council for Graduate Medical Education; Adjunct Professor, Yale University; Professor Emeritus, Mayo Clinic; and Professor Emeritus, University of Minnesota

# The Long Arc of Training
## Six Stories of Aspiring Doctors

Dorene F. Balmer

University of Toronto Press
Toronto Buffalo London

© Dorene Balmer 2026
Toronto Buffalo London
utppublishing.com

ISBN 978-1-4875-6559-6 (paper)  ISBN 978-1-4875-6562-6 (EPUB)
ISBN 978-1-4875-6561-9 (PDF)

---

**Library and Archives Canada Cataloguing in Publication**

Title: The long arc of training : six stories of aspiring doctors / Dorene Balmer.
Names: Balmer, Dorene, author.
Description: Includes bibliographical references and index.
Identifiers: Canadiana (print) 20250296047 | Canadiana (ebook) 2025029611X | ISBN 9781487565596 (paper) | ISBN 9781487565619 (PDF) | ISBN 9781487565626 (EPUB)
Subjects: LCSH: Physicians – Training of. | LCSH: Medical education.
Classification: LCC R690 .B35 2026 | DDC 610.69 – dc23

---

Cover design: Georgie Proctor
Cover image: Shutterstock.com / alya_haciyeva

We wish to acknowledge the land on which the University of Toronto Press operates. This land is the traditional territory of the Wendat, the Anishnaabeg, the Haudenosaunee, the Métis, and the Mississaugas of the Credit First Nation.

University of Toronto Press acknowledges the financial support of the Government of Canada, the Canada Council for the Arts, and the Ontario Arts Council, an agency of the Government of Ontario, for its publishing activities.

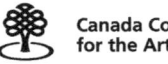
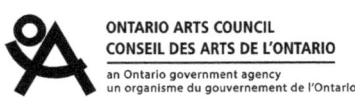
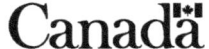

# Contents

*Acknowledgments* vii

Introduction: Blake's Story About Transformation 1

1 Eliza's Story About Socialization 29

2 Alan's Story About Agency 55

3 Niki's Story About Balance 82

4 Krista's Story About Emotion 108

5 Tim's Story About Comfort 135

6 The End of the Arc 158

*A Note to Aspiring Doctors* 171
*Notes* 175
*Index* 183

# Acknowledgments

This book has been a labor of love for well over a decade. It began as a research study and grew into something I could not have imagined at the start – a work of narrative nonfiction that tells the stories of six remarkable doctors as they moved through medical school, residency, fellowship and into clinical practice. I owe thanks to many people who have walked alongside me, as I walked alongside the participants.

**To the participants**
First and foremost, my deepest gratitude goes to the six participants themselves. You are long-suffering, brave, and kind. My hope is that this book offers something of value back to you, and to all the doctors who come after you.

**To my mentors and colleagues**

To Dr. Olson Pook – you helped me see the possibilities of this book long before I did: a project rooted in rigorous research yet destined to live beyond the academy. Your coaching, creativity, and diligence gave me the courage to share my work in an unfamiliar genre and to believe in myself as a writer.

When I was ready to give up on the project after nine years and multiple manuscript rejections, Dr. Pim Teunissen reminded me that this work was ahead of its time – that the space for narrative nonfiction in health professions education had not yet caught up. Your encouragement kept me going, and your leadership continues to inspire me to imagine a field that can embrace scholarship that challenges the status quo.

This book would not exist without the support of Dr. Boyd Richards and Dr. Mike Devlin. You were both there from the beginning, back when I thought I was simply researching how medical students learn health system science. Boyd – rarely does a mentor-turned-friend stay the course for more than a decade. You did, and you are one of a kind. Mike – your thoughtful readings and deep insights into the long arc of training enriched this project in countless ways.

To my critical friend, Dr. A. Emiko Blalock – what a gift it has been to share this path with you. Our conversations, shifting seamlessly between personal updates and constructive critique, always left me feeling supported. Our shared passion for longitudinal qualitative research – and our friendship – are treasures I carry with me.

**To my professional home**
Throughout the length of this study, I benefited from the support of colleagues at the medical centers where I worked. I am especially grateful to Dr. Daniel West, Dr. Joseph St. Geme III and the Department of Pediatrics at the Perelman School of Medicine at the University of Pennsylvania. The generosity extended through a Distinguished Endowed Chair made this book possible.

**To my editorial team and publisher**
Bringing this project into the world would not have been possible without the editorial team at University of Toronto Press. I am grateful for their belief in the book and for the care they brought to every stage of its production.

**To my family**
Finally, to my partner, River Dunavin, and my nephew, Josh Balmer – thank you for supporting me through every high and low of this twelve-year process. I could not have done this without you.

And to all who made space for this work along the way – thank you. This book is, in the end, about journeys. I am grateful to everyone who has been part of mine.

INTRODUCTION

# Blake's Story About Transformation

Tell all the truth but tell it slant —
Success in Circuit lies
Too bright for our infirm Delight
The Truth's superb surprise
As Lightning to the Children eased
With explanation kind
The Truth must dazzle gradually
Or every man be blind —
— Emily Dickinson (1263)

## Introduction: "The Truth must dazzle gradually"

It was the middle of winter. Boston was frigid and streets were sloppy with wet snow. It seemed the only reason people were out on this Sunday evening was to go to one of the many coffee shops dotting the neighborhoods. Blake was in one when I called, working through all the emails that had accumulated over a busy stretch of clinical service. He was halfway through his first year of residency, the period of medical training after medical school. The first year (also called internship) was the most onerous. Rounds – when the medical team methodically visits each and every patient assigned to their care – started before daybreak, which meant Blake arrived at the hospital even earlier to prepare. His clinical service responsibilities ended well after dusk. Sometimes they didn't end until the next day when he was on call and worked a twenty-four-hour shift. Blake had anticipated long hours. But what he did not anticipate was how life-changing medical training could be:

> A part of the training that people don't realize is how transformative it can be. It's not like a regular job where you are just learning things. People who go through this process kind of find themselves, or at least learn how to be a physician and learn about new parts of themselves. It's more the divide between job and profession. I think most people who have been through medical training will feel that the way they come out is not the way that they started.

It wasn't like Blake had started medical school with a clear picture of his future self that was then shattered and rebuilt from the ground up. That wasn't the transformation. In fact, he started medical school feeling a little envious of his classmates who knew since they were children that they wanted to be pediatricians or surgeons: "I was sort of jealous of how certain they were, how confident they were in their career decision." When Blake talked about transformation in medical training, he was referring to something much more nuanced than a career choice. He was referring to constructing an identity – a sense of self – as a doctor and how subtly that happened through time:

> I think doctors tend to see themselves differently after a while, and I don't mean that in an egotistical way. You don't stop being a doctor. Even when I'm on vacation, even when I'm out at dinner – and it's happened to me where I'm on a plane and someone called out, "Is there a doctor on board?" I don't think I realized, or people realize that you don't stop being a doctor … It's part of the transformation that people don't think about.

I was talking to Blake because I'm a social scientist in medical education and interested in understanding how medical students eventually become doctors – not the obvious process of passing high-stakes licensing exams and graduating from medical school, but how they shape and reshape their sense of self over the long course of their training. Blake's point about the transformation doctors experience is well put, but what interested me in what he said was how people don't think about *the transformative process*. What did he mean, and why was that the case? Blake's story about his own high-order transformation is fascinating in its own right but also sets the stage for more detailed investigations of the different transformations the other doctors in this book shared with me.

In this chapter and the ones that follow, I curate the stories told to me by six aspiring doctors that illuminate the transformations they experienced in medical training (and since every curator is also a storyteller, I've come to identify as such, despite my ties to academia). While television shows like *ER* and *Grey's Anatomy* dramatically portray that transformation, these real-life narratives reveal something far more nuanced: the gradual, often invisible process of becoming a doctor. For current doctors reading these pages, these stories might echo their own journeys through medical training, or they might unveil journeys that unfolded quite differently. For those considering medicine as a career, these stories offer authentic glimpses into the evolving and nuanced ways medical trainees construct their identities. And given the general public's unquenchable thirst for entertaining stories about doctors, I suspect these stories will strike a chord with those readers as well.

But these stories serve another critical purpose: they challenge how we study the transformation of medical students into full-fledged doctors. While the doctors in these pages consistently describe becoming a physician as a deeply personal, dynamic, and nonlinear process, scholars in medical education have almost always relied on snapshots rather than follow the long arc of the transformation. It seems too obvious to say, but if we don't study the process of becoming a doctor – from start to finish as it unfolds in the lives of individual trainees – we will miss critical aspects of how medical students transform into doctors. Yet if we slow down and take a closer look at the transformative process as it occurs, we will be amazed and dazzled at what we discover.

## "Tell all the truth": The need to consider time

For too long, the field of medical education has tried to tell all the truth about medical training but wound up only telling partial truths based on cross-sectional data collected at a single point in time. But a complex phenomenon like the transformative process that Blake talked about isn't something that happens over days or weeks or even a year. Watching that process unfold requires walking alongside aspiring doctors to discover how, where, and why such profound transformation happens. Although cross-sectional studies are typically more feasible and cost-effective than longitudinal ones, what they reveal is different from the unfolding insights generated when you return time and again to the same participants. Telling partial truth(s) comes at a cost. Lost in cross-sectional studies is the long arc of time: how the manifold past informs the dynamic present and shapes the future.

Moreover, the field of medical education has wound up telling partial truths based on data derived from recollections, asking trainees to remember "back when." Researchers certainly can ask participants to recall their past, thereby capturing their memory of events, but those recollections will always be contextualized in the reality of the present. Memory has a way of distorting the past. Robert Waldinger, a psychiatrist and director of the Harvard

Study of Adult Development – the longest-running ongoing longitudinal study – explained the limitations of recollections this way:

> Pictures of entire lives – of the choices that people make and how those choices work out for them – those pictures are almost impossible to get. Most of what we know about human life we know from asking people to remember the past, and as we know, hindsight is anything but 20/20. We forget vast amounts of what happens to us in life. And sometimes, memory is downright creative. But what if we could watch entire lives as they unfold through time?[1]

Watching how medical trainees transform through time is exactly what I did with the six doctors profiled in the pages that follow. A longitudinal approach reveals how, over the course of medical training, aspiring doctors tap into their past, situate themselves in the present, and project themselves into the future. In essence, a longitudinal approach hinges on time. But thinking about time as only a series of discrete events in time (A then B then C) is far too simplistic. What participants saw and knew at one point in time could be seen and known in a radically different way a few years later. Time is a series of interconnected events flowing into one another. Even so, there are moments when time seemed to stand still. As one of the doctors in this book explained, "What's hard about the transition from one year of residency to the next is when you don't feel like you are transitioning. You're just in it. It doesn't even feel like you're moving." But move through time they did.

I've come to believe that telling a longitudinal story about medical training is a way of getting closer to the truth, at least as experienced by the doctors in this book. We learn things we would not have discovered otherwise because time teaches us that nothing on the surface, or in the moment, is exactly as it seems. A crawling, recursive, and deliberate yet simultaneously open-ended approach affords us opportunities to gain a deeper understanding of the transformative process of becoming a doctor. Blake and others in this book found that reflecting on their own journeys and narrating their own growth was revealing in ways even they did not anticipate. "I don't know that I would have been as introspective about things," Blake admitted. "Answering questions that I've never really thought about has to have had some effect over time."

## "But tell it slant": The work of transformation

Blake's comment about transformation points to an ongoing process that happens in and through time. And yet, the field of medical education has erected walls between phases of training and sees the transitions between them as particularly transformative. For example, it is generally accepted that moving from medical school to residency is transformational for doctors-in-training. But a longitudinal approach reveals that what resonates as a transformational moment for one trainee may not resonate for another. In Blake's case, the transformation wasn't cast in terms of the transition between phases, but in terms of celebrated rites of passage. Donning a white coat in his first year of medical school was transformative for him because, in his mind, it distinguished him from patients:

> It has been a really good experience to go into the hospital and learn how to interact with patients, how to take a history and do a physical exam and feel like I have some practical skills. As I start my second year of medical school, I'm starting to feel more comfortable wearing my white coat now and carrying it around.

What a longitudinal approach revealed was that Blake's transformation didn't end there. He wore a short white coat as a medical student, which was just a springboard to the longer white coat he would wear in residency. For Blake, moving between coats was part of his transformation:

> Part of the learning curve was the gain in confidence when wearing the longer white coat and seeing myself as a doctor and responding when someone calls you "doctor." Whereas before, when I was wearing a shorter white coat as a medical student, I was following patients and I was involved but did not feel as acutely responsible for every aspect of their care. You're there and you're part of their care, but ultimately it is someone else's responsibility to make sure things get done. But now it's all on me.

For another doctor in this book, a major transformation happened between her first and second years of residency when she started to take on a supervisory role: "The transition from first year to second year of residency has done more to set me on the path to who I will ultimately be as an attending than the jump from medical school to residency."

This book then is an attempt to provide an intimate look into the transformative process of becoming a doctor – not by offering snapshots of different trainees at various phases or presenting their recollections – but by centering the stories of real-life aspiring doctors as those stories unfolded. Their narratives reveal flashbacks of what they learned about themselves and what they had gone through, and foreshadowings of how much further they had to go to be the doctors they wanted to be.

## "With explanation kind": The path to becoming a doctor

Understanding the phases of medical education is a necessary first step to grasping the particulars of any journey to becoming a doctor. Just as familiarity with military terminology such as NCO (noncommissioned officer) and ROE (rules of engagement), the distinctions between being a private, lieutenant, or major, and the pathways to joining the military (enlisting, military academy, or Reserve Officers Training Corps/ROTC) is helpful to understand a soldier's career path, so too will a basic familiarity with the terminology, distinctions, and pathways to becoming a physician or surgeon aid in grasping the details in the stories that follow.

In the United States, doctors receive more training over more years than almost any other profession. In terms of schooling, you can become a police officer or electrician without a college degree. You need a college degree to be a teacher or engineer. And you need a postgraduate degree to become a lawyer. Yet doctors not only go to college for four years but also attend medical school for another four. Then they stick around for between three to seven years after medical school to get additional on-the-job training in residency. After that, some even do several years of subspecialized training in fellowship.

For many would-be medical students, undergraduate life is a relentless whirlwind of academic rigor and intense competition. Each day is packed with lectures on topics like organic chemistry and human physiology, followed by laboratory sessions demanding acute attention to detail. The pressure to excel is inescapable, given that grades become part of your medical school application. Aside from studying, there's the constant juggling of extracurricular activities, research, and volunteer hours – which (as we shall see) are all crucial elements for a compelling medical school application. While some trainees go straight from college to medical school, others take a year off to gain research or clinical experience. Some even have gone into other careers only to decide to return to college and complete prerequisite courses for medical school. Regardless of their path, all must apply to medical school, a grueling process that involves filling out applications, submitting transcripts, requesting letters of recommendation, being interviewed, and, of course, preparing for and scoring well on the MCAT (Medical College Admissions Test).

Once accepted into medical school, the academic rigor and competition don't just continue but ramp up even more. When the doctors in this book were starting medical school, most curricula were designed to provide a heavy dose of classroom instruction in the first eighteen to twenty-four months (also called the pre-clerkship phase). After memorizing an overwhelming volume of facts spanning the basic medical sciences, medical students move out of the classroom and into the clerkship year. Clerkships are required clinical rotations in specialties such as internal medicine, surgery, neurology, psychiatry, pediatrics, obstetrics and gynecology, and primary care. Rotations occur in real-life clinical learning environments and typically last four to six weeks. The clerkship year can feel like a revolving door: by the time medical students feel at ease on one rotation, it's time to move on to another. On these rotations, students join a medical team, consisting of residents (doctors who have completed medical school and moved on to training within a specialty), fellows (doctors who have completed residency and chosen to study a subspecialty) and attendings (full-fledged physicians or surgeons in charge of the medical team). Tasks assigned to medical students are quite limited, and they may feel like an obstacle to the team's efficiency in patient care. Nonetheless, students are legitimate members of the team and expected to engage with patients as they explore a variety of specialties. Although residents, fellows, and attendings informally teach medical students while providing care, there is relatively little in the way of formal instruction compared to the pre-clerkship phase.

In the final phase of medical school, students complete sub-internships, which are more intense, compulsory clinical rotations. Sub-internships could be in the same setting as clerkships or in settings like a surgical intensive care unit, a research-oriented inpatient psychiatric unit, or a pediatric oncology ward. In this final phase, students also do elective rotations in specialties they are considering for residency. But first they have to answer some specific questions about their future careers in medicine: What type of patient encounters are they drawn toward: acute or chronic? How much direct patient contact do they want? What kinds of procedural skills are required? What type of lifestyle can they anticipate? How does the salary compare with any educational loans they need to repay? But before they move on from medical school, they must pass the high-stakes United States Medical Licensing Examinations (USMLE), then interview and apply for residency. Only then are medical students matched to a residency program via a complex mathematical algorithm that aligns the training preferences of medical students with the preferences of residency programs.

While graduates of medical school are newly minted doctors, training is not over. Residency is an intense, hands-on phase of training in a medical or surgical specialty that follows medical school. Residencies typically are located at teaching hospitals and vary in focus (for example, general surgery versus a more specialized surgery like orthopedic surgery), in orientation (for example, more clinical versus more research), and in length (for example, three years for pediatrics versus four years for anesthesia). Like medical school, residencies consist of rotations and immersive learning experiences in different areas of clinical practice. For instance, an internal medicine resident might rotate through cardiology and endocrinology while an anesthesia resident might rotate through internal and emergency medicine.

Although there are attempts to on-board residents, residency is still very much baptism by fire. The feeling of being overwhelmed returns, only this time, instead of the initial crush of biomedical science in medical school, it's the crush of patient care. In addition, what is expected of residents is different from what is expected of medical students in terms of levels of responsibility. As residents gain experience, their supervisors (who are attending physicians or surgeons) progressively extend more responsibility to them. In medical school, every moment was potentially a teaching moment, with a resident, fellow, or an attending nearby. But now residents are the ones overseeing medical students, while at the same time being supervised (albeit more indirectly) by senior residents, fellows, or attendings. And then there's the money: Unlike medical students who pay medical school tuition, residents receive a moderate salary for the patient care they provide. Finally, if the hours are long in medical school, they are even longer in residency – so much so that in 2003, the Accreditation Council for Graduate Medical Education established a maximum eighty-hour work week and reduced the length of shifts to no longer than thirty hours.[2] But setting limits on work hours does not limit the intensity of those work hours. Blake spoke revealingly about his own experience and ensuing doubts: "Being a resident is hard, and there are definitely times when I think to myself, is this really what I want to do with my life?"

Residents in ACGME-accredited programs are expected to perform in ways that align with their developmental stage across six core competencies: medical knowledge, patient care, interpersonal communication, professionalism, practice-based learning and improvement (learning from one's own practice and external evidence), and systems-based practice (being aware of the larger context of healthcare and being able to tap into local healthcare resources).[3] While residents gain competence largely through doing the work of patient care alongside senior residents, fellows, and attendings, there are also formal educational sessions like morning reports, grand rounds, and noon conferences.

Upon graduation from residency, residents are eligible to take their specialty board examination and become board-certified in their specialty. Board certification goes above and beyond state licensing and represents a commitment to continuously expanding knowledge in a specialty. At this point, they can enter general practice as a general pediatrician, a general anesthesiologist, or a general surgeon. However, if they want to practice as a subspecialist (e.g., a cardio-thoracic surgeon or pediatric endocrinologist), they must complete subspecialty fellowship training. Those who choose to do a fellowship gain even more specialized knowledge and skills, such as advanced surgical techniques, diagnostic procedures, or forms of treatment. Like residencies, fellowships vary in length and orientation, with some having dedicated research time and research requirements and others being more clinically oriented. As revealed in some of the stories in this book, fellowships are not required for general practice, but those who choose to stay in academic medicine, where patient care, medical education, and research intersect, often complete a fellowship.

## "Success in Circuit lies": My journey to longitudinal qualitative research

The chapters in this book showcase the stories of aspiring doctors, with Blake's story setting the stage for them. But understanding how I came to witness, curate, and tell the stories I did will help explain the evolution of this book and the insights that I discovered. In contrast to the prescribed path to becoming a doctor, there were no direct paths into medical education. In fact, for me there was no direct path into academia. I'm the daughter of a farmer, a first-generation college graduate who found her way from serving food as a waitress after high school to studying food and nutrition in college and becoming a registered dietitian. There are different career options for those who study nutrition. I was drawn to hospital-based work because it satisfied my thirst for continual learning and desire to stay up to date in my practice. So I entered the professional world at a large children's hospital affiliated with a research-intensive university in the Northeast United States.

I am admittedly not a medical doctor like the ones in this book, but I, too, started my professional life in the setting of academic medicine. Many of my colleagues were medical trainees. While I thoroughly enjoyed working as a registered dietitian and being part of a multidisciplinary care team, I was passionate about education. So rather than pursuing a master's degree in nutrition, I went on to pursue a master's degree in education. I worked at the hospital during the day and then drove an hour to take evening classes at a small private university. Like most other graduate students, I went to a classroom, took semester-long courses, had a single instructor, followed a syllabus, and completed predetermined assignments.

Meanwhile, the medical trainees with whom I worked during the day were in "clinical classrooms" – busy hospital wards filled with very sick patients. They had no semesters but rotated through different units a month at a time. Instead of a single instructor who saw their progress over several months, they had multiple attendings who supervised their work one week at a time. They had no formal syllabus; learning was "on the fly," dependent on the number and types of patients who needed care, and their "assignments" were not readings or papers but real-life patient care. This is all to say that I graduated not only with a master's degree but also an acute awareness that their training was not at all like mine.

The same thirst for learning that drew me to hospital-based work drew me to do a PhD. My firsthand experience with residents in clinical classrooms drove my doctoral research agenda. I had no interest in studying the deliberate, formal medical education that was mandated by the ACGME and intentionally structured. What interested me was what and how residents could learn in unpredictable, messy, and demanding clinical environments.

While my professional training was different from that of the doctors I studied, we had one thing in common: we learned that research within the realm of academic medicine entailed systematic study of the physical and natural world through observation, hypothesis testing and experimentation, and generation of objective and verifiable evidence. Unsurprisingly, when it came to designing my doctoral research, I really struggled. This way of thinking about research could not accommodate the kinds of research questions I was asking about clinical classrooms that couldn't be moved to a lab or manipulated in situ.

I'll be forever grateful for a course I took that introduced me to qualitative research – the systematic study of social realities through understanding how people experience their world and welcoming the researcher into the research endeavor. I felt like I had discovered a treasure chest that had sunk to the bottom of the sea in academic medicine. When I unlocked it, I found just what I needed to answer my research questions. Specifically, I came upon ethnography, a methodology with roots in anthropology that entails close, prolonged observation and engagement in a natural setting to understand how social groups navigate their world. I would end up doing an ethnographic study in my doctoral research, looking at things like apprenticeship learning and the pedagogical power of physician role models in an outpatient pediatric setting.[4] I did another ethnographic study in my postdoctoral research, exploring how residents implicitly learned the formal curriculum during hands-on training in an inpatient pediatric ward.[5] As much as I loved doing ethnography, what left a lasting impression on me was the enduring research relationships. I was hooked.

## "Infirm Delight": How this book came to be

My first faculty position was in an education support center at a medical school in a city neighboring the one where I worked as a registered dietitian. This medical school was launching a new program for students interested in health systems improvement. They would experience the same pre-clerkship curriculum as students in the traditional program, but they would have a different, integrated clerkship experience. Rather than rotating through specialties, they would follow a panel of patients at a different hospital for a full year, across all the required specialties.[6] In my investigator mind, this new program created a unique opportunity for research. I envisioned myself doing an ethnographic study that explored how medical students learn, implicitly and explicitly, about health systems by virtue of being in two different hospitals – one at the "mother ship" in the city and the other in a rural area.

My colleague Dr. Boyd Richards and I partnered in the early part of this study; Boyd brought years of practical experience in medical education, and I brought enthusiasm and qualitative research skills. We launched the study in fall of 2010, enrolling 9 out of the 10 students in the new program and 14 of the 150 students in the traditional program. I interviewed students twice in their first year of medical school (midway and at the end) and did a third round of interviews midway through their second year, right before they started their clerkships.

What I recognized as exceptional was my growing relationships with students who would faithfully respond to my requests for another interview. I never had less than an 80 per cent participation rate – and most times it was 100 per cent. What was even more remarkable was that I started to hear students say things like, "I've never told anyone this before." But doing ethnography while having a full-time job as a faculty member proved to be quite different from doing ethnography as a doctoral student or a postdoc fellow. I just couldn't commit the time to the kind of observation that would be necessary to address my original research question. I thought my study was an ethnography, but I was wrong.

Nevertheless, I was tenacious. Boyd's encouragement matched with my persistence was reason enough to continue with the interviews and drop the observational arm of the study. I did a fourth round of interviews in the summer of 2012 when students were nearing the end of their clerkships. I did a fifth round of interviews when students were in their final year of medical school and sitting with considerable uncertainty because they had not yet been matched to a residency program. I thought the study would end here as graduation from medical school seemed like a logical ending point. But I was wrong again.

At the end of 2014, most of the participants had graduated from medical school and moved on to residency. I myself had moved to another institution. But when several students asked about the possibility of continuing our conversations, I didn't have the heart to say no. The first inkling that the research might go on longer came from a remark Blake made: "You're probably one of the only people that I've really reflected on my medical school experience with. I appreciate your dedication, and as long as you're still willing to keep doing it, I'll be willing to keep going." I started to write my first manuscript, and in doing background reading for it, I uncovered a substantive gap in the literature – there were no studies that purposefully followed the same group of students from medical school into residency. I was astonished. I thought surely others would have walked alongside students-turned-residents. I was wrong again.

But there was a problem. After five rounds of interviews with over twenty students, I was drowning in qualitative data. I knew I couldn't keep up with everyone. To manage the workload, I narrowed the sample to six. Two were headed to pediatric residencies, which aligned with my work in a children's hospital. Two other students wanted to continue – one headed to surgery and one to anesthesia. I asked another student who was doing a surgical residency and another doing an anesthesia residency if they would be interested and willing to continue. Both agreed. So I had my group of six, split evenly between males and females, with one identifying as Hispanic and one as Southeast Asian. They had other diverse characteristics. Two had been in the new program and did their integrated clerkship at a hospital in a rural area. Two took a year out of medical school to complete a master's degree. Among the six, two eventually opted to leave academic medicine. From a personal standpoint, over the course of the study, five got married and four started families.

When Boyd and I began the study, all participants were first-year medical students going through the same pre-clerkship experience at the same medical school. But what began as a lockstep progression went off the rails when participants moved into residency. Each went to different residencies of varying length: two were in three-year residencies, two were in four-year residencies, one was in a five-year residency, and one in a six-year residency. Two went into general practice right after residency. The other four extended their training and did a fellowship, lasting from one to three years. But more substantive than different lengths of training were different ways they were socialized into their specialty. Two became surgeons – a specialty so distinct from medicine that its practitioners take a title other than doctor. Two entered the surgery-related, procedure-rich field of anesthesia, which required skillful use of one's hands. The other two did pediatric residencies, which are stereotypically the "soft and fuzzy" opposite of surgeons.

What Blake said at the beginning of this chapter about medical training – that "the way that you come out is not the way that you started" – could have applied to my own transformation as a researcher in medical education. Around this time, I read work by Johnny Saldaña and realized that what I was doing had a name – longitudinal qualitative research.[7] Engaging with the same participants in research over long periods of time requires a leap into the unknown. This time, I was absolutely right.

Longitudinal researchers are not exactly sure how long the study will last, where it will lead, or what they will find. In doing longitudinal qualitative research, I had to reconceptualize the phenomenon that I was studying. An overreliance on formal theories bogged me down and detracted from the stories I wanted to tell. When I spoke to participants on a six to twelve month basis, I would routinely share things they had said over the years and ask them, "Where are you with that now?" They were responding to their earlier selves and updating their understanding. With this type of recursive interviewing, I realized that the participants were narrating their growth, much like I am narrating my own now. Tellingly, none of the topics I cover in subsequent chapters was derived directly from interview questions I asked. But all participants spoke to these topics in some way, shape, or form as they answered my main interview questions: tell me about a peak experience or learning highlight since we last spoke; what does that experience say about what's important to you? What have you learned about yourself as a doctor? What lessons have you learned about what it will take to be a doctor in today's society? Is there anything else you think I should know about but didn't ask?

As the years ticked by, I realized that if nobody had followed the same cohort of medical students through residency, then no one had followed the same cohort from medical school into practice. My participants were game, so we continued until everyone was in practice – a total of twelve years. One of the participants was in training for twelve consecutive years. Others were in training for seven to eight years, and so their stories include the first few years of practice as physicians or surgeons.

This book centers their stories, which I came closer and closer to understanding with each round of interviews. I avoided overanalyzing them in terms of theory; to do so runs the risk of jeopardizing the integrity of the stories told by the aspiring doctors in this book. In fact, as the stories that follow attest, what I observed oftentimes challenges or at least recasts the accepted wisdom issuing from existing literature. To stay grounded in the power of narrative, I use lines from a different poem for each chapter that reveal in their own way – like Emily Dickinson's "Tell all the truth but tell it slant" (1263) – what I found when tracing the progression through their narrative.

## "The Truth's superb surprise": What their stories revealed

In five subsequent chapters, I tell the stories of five medical students on their journey to becoming attending physicians or surgeons. In so doing, I give form to their experience and to the complex process of becoming a doctor. Through time, salient subject matter or themes were discussed over and over, even if how they talked about them evolved (for example, some dimensions of transformation started out as "doing the work of a doctor" in medical school but shifted to "being a doctor" in residency). These themes became the focus of the subsequent chapters. To keep individual storylines intact, I showcase one participant who serves as an illustrative example of the theme in any given chapter. But as the themes transcended individual narratives, the voices of the other doctors appear across all chapters.

The stories in this book are not fictional. They are not derived from composite characters created to represent common experiences in medical education. Instead, they are real people, and the stories reflect unique journeys through the long arc of medical training. By focusing on these individual accounts, I hope to offer a nuanced and personalized view of some of the less-recognized and taken-for-granted parts of the journey to becoming a doctor.

From Eliza in Chapter 1, we learn how the social structures of elite medical schools (which I define as those that have disproportional control over or access to resources like funding for biomedical research) can surprisingly narrow one's career options because only some career choices are perceived as "pure medicine." Since childhood, Eliza had her eyes set on becoming a doctor and cared about going to reputable schools. At the same time, she had big aspirations to improve healthcare for children in underserved parts of the world by intervening at a health systems level – something that fell outside the scope of elite medicine's ambitions. Torn between both, she initially opted for a "road less taken" and completed a business degree despite the expectation to study biomedical science. But Eliza surprised even herself when she fell in love with surgery, even though her chosen field wasn't particularly accommodating of her adjacent interest in health systems science. Contrary to her assumption that getting into an elite medical school would open doors, Eliza's journey to becoming a doctor was marked by unexpected tensions stemming from the doors she wanted to enter but which "pure medicine" seemingly closed.

Alan is the poster child of the nontraditional medical school applicant from whom we learn in Chapter 2 about agency – not the expectation to take initiative or agency bounded by a particular context, but a temporally embedded process of social engagement. A former pianist and self-taught software developer, Alan went to medical school a bit later in life. He was cognizant of the pressure to "do something big" but was also aware of his need to fit his career into the larger whole of his life, to juggle his need for creativity and to support his family with the demands of a career in medicine. We see him pursue anesthesiology and make career choices that run counter to what was expected of him, like choosing to work in private practice. The thread of agency runs through his story as he routinely considers saying yes, but graciously says no.

From Niki in Chapter 3 we learn that burnout can be usefully understood as the lack of balance between meaning derived from work as a doctor and the demands of the workplace. Balance is much bigger and more holistic than the absence of burnout. Dead set on obstetrics and gynecology when she started medical school, Niki's certainty was shattered when she realized that she actually hated doing surgical procedures, which was a big part of obstetrics and gynecology. Throughout her story, Niki pulled on earlier life experiences to recalibrate in response to different stressors. She found potential for balance in pediatrics, so she completed her pediatric residency and went straight to work in pediatric primary care. Across a series of unsettling events,

Niki tweaked her career goals and navigated career decisions in ways that prioritized her young and growing family.

From Krista in Chapter 4 we learn about how the "emotion work" doctors engage in goes much further than just being empathic. Enamored with role-playing games like Dungeons and Dragons and the emotional rollercoaster that players experienced, Krista was all in when it came to connecting with patients and being part of their medical dramas. Things changed when she got into pediatric residency, and the emotional rollercoaster was no longer a game but part of her everyday life. Over the course of residency, a two-year stint as a frontline provider, and a three-year neonatology fellowship, Krista discovered that equally important to becoming a doctor was discovering that — despite what the literature reported — the empathy she had for her patients didn't actually decline and that rules about not catering to public display of emotions could be broken.

We discover the central role of "feeling comfortable" as an internal marker of progress from Tim in Chapter 5. Although often dismissed as merely a subjective emotion with no place in competency-based medical education, "feeling comfortable" was what Tim routinely returned to as he moved through the multiple stages of surgical residency and fellowship. Just like other doctors in this book, he needed to feel confident in his knowledge and skills. But feeling comfortable was a step beyond confidence. It was adapting to the unexpected and still delivering safe and effective patient care.

Blake is the main contributor to this introductory chapter. His story provides a high-level commentary about the transformative process of becoming a doctor – the repeated farewell to his former self and embracing who he was becoming. Subsequent chapters delve into different specific manifestations of that transformative process. Like the others in this book, Blake makes cameos in the other chapters. But by way of this introductory chapter, Blake shows us that becoming a doctor was much more than just a career choice; it was an unfolding process.

## Conclusion: "As Lightning"

The doctors in this book eagerly engaged in this study from the start of medical school, unaware (as was I) of what lay ahead. They willingly engaged as medical training became more intense. They openly engaged as they grappled with weighty career decisions entangled with their personal lives. They graciously engaged as years went on and I struggled to figure out how best to disseminate their stories. In the end, each chapter in the book represents one individual's journey to becoming a doctor. These journeys, let alone the practice of medicine, can be dramatic, so it's not surprising that most people learn about medical training through the guise of fictional characters in series like *ER* or *Grey's Anatomy*. But the stories that follow are not fiction. In their diversity and authenticity they offer a compelling collage of what it is like for real people to become doctors.

While I am the author of this book, it is the words of the aspiring doctors that take up much of the pages that follow. I witnessed their stories, generated from serial, recursive interviews, and conferred form onto their experiences so that others can learn from them.[8] In focusing on specific subject matter within these stories, I acknowledge that I guide readers to attend to some aspects of the long arc of training but not others. And each participant has their own personal narrative that would undoubtedly be somewhat different from the story I tell in this book. While I used pseudonyms and avoided sharing details that might be identifying, they readily recognized themselves and their experience in the words that follow.[9]

My highest hope for this book is that it addresses a singular curiosity of the doctors portrayed on these pages, all of whom wondered what would have changed for them, if, before they went into medicine, they had read a book about different types of doctors sharing their transformations as medical trainees. I hope the stories will help aspiring doctors know what they might anticipate and what they might overlook if they don't consider the long arc of training – what they might strive for and what they might let go of. I hope this book will give current doctors a glimpse of themselves in these stories. I hope it will also inform medical school faculty who shape the learning and the careers of trainees, sometimes more powerfully (and sometimes less powerfully) than they know. I hope these stories inspire scholars in the field of medical education to broaden their methodological horizons and consider longitudinal qualitative research. And finally, I hope these stories satisfy and stimulate the minds of general readers outside the medical profession; may they discover that the "lightning strike of truth" can be just as (if not more) intriguing than fiction.

CHAPTER 1

# Eliza's Story About Socialization

Two roads diverged in a yellow wood,
And sorry I could not travel both
And be one traveler, long I stood
And looked down one as far as I could
To where it bent in the undergrowth;

Then took the other, as just as fair,
And having perhaps the better claim,
Because it was grassy and wanted wear;
Though as for that the passing there
Had worn them really about the same,

And both that morning equally lay
In leaves no step had trodden black.
Oh, I kept the first for another day!

> Yet knowing how way leads on to way,
> I doubted if I should ever come back.
>
> I shall be telling this with a sigh
> Somewhere ages and ages hence:
> Two roads diverged in a wood, and I—
> I took the one less traveled by,
> And that has made all the difference.
> – Robert Frost, "The Road Not Taken"

## Introduction: "Two roads diverged"

When Eliza and I spoke over Zoom during her year as a fellow in a surgical subspecialty, she was sitting on a porch, her back to the park in the distance. The fact that trees and not skyscrapers dotted the landscape behind her was a tipoff that she was no longer in her native New York City. The only thing that retained a sense of the harried quality of her hometown was Eliza herself. Small for her size, she carried the energy of the city wherever she went.

Being a doctor was something Eliza wanted to do for as long as she could remember. The route she took to get there was somewhat atypical – studying political science in college and taking a gap year in the middle of medical school to get a business degree. Nonetheless, one thing that she had in common with the other doctors in this book was her desire to be the best doctor she could be – and that meant studying at one of the best medical schools. In her mind, like many in medicine, "best" meant elite. Attending an elite university for college and then an elite medical school were central to developing an academic pedigree – a lineage that follows alma maters and not bloodlines.[1] The aspiring doctors in this book, all graduates of the same highly ranked medical school, acknowledged that academic pedigree worked to their advantage: "Going to [this medical school] basically guaranteed that I could do whatever I wanted," Niki remarked. "No doors would be closed to me." When the doctors in this book were applying for residency and going after jobs, their pedigree in terms of the medical school they graduated from mattered. Reminiscent of Frost's poem, pedigree would lead them down one road but not another.

More than the other doctors in this book, Eliza was candid about the value she placed on her academic pedigree. "I care a lot about reputation and name recognition. We have these metrics that we use to grade success, and mine has always been getting into the best schools."

Whether reputation and name recognition are valid metrics to grade success as a doctor is a topic of ongoing debate, and the popular medical school rankings are under fire.[2] Nonetheless, there is a pervasive belief in medicine and in society at large that going to an elite medical school predicts success in the medical profession. What counts as an elite medical school is largely determined by national rankings that heavily weigh the school's ability to obtain federal funding for biomedical research, even though research funding may have little bearing on patient outcomes. Eliza admitted her metrics were controversial. But her belief that academic pedigree was a metric for success had ramifications, to the tune of her turning down a scholarship to attend a lower ranked medical school in favor of paying full tuition at an elite medical school.

What medical students like Eliza didn't foresee when they started their training at an elite medical school were the downstream career consequences of being attracted to academic pedigree. Many of these consequences were quite positive: students graduated not only with a coveted diploma but also with other resources like social connections that positioned them for future success in medicine. But staying on an elite trajectory in medicine had another consequence: it could narrow career choices. Trajectories were shaped by elite medicine's professional norms and expectations that deemed some career choices acceptable but not others. Just six months out of medical school, Tim talked about the tunnel vision he had as a medical student – the kind of narrow perspective that limits the career alternatives that students consider and pigeonholes the kinds of careers they pursue:

> In terms of your career aspirations, the only model you see is a highly funded academic institution. There is the prestige in terms of gaining the residencies and ultimately the fellowships and employments that will mirror the models you see. Elite medical schools like this one prepare you well, or at least guide you to that model. But you come away with certain pernicious conceptions – or at least I did. You see a research-intensive, academic institution, and that is what you want to replicate in residency, in fellowship, and as an attending.

This chapter explores the consequences of socialization into medicine – learning the ropes of becoming a doctor – at an elite medical school on how students built their careers. Speaking of academia at large, sociologist Shamus Khan defines elites as those who have disproportional control over or access to valued resources.[3] In line with this definition, elite medical schools have disproportional control over or access to resources like federal funding for biomedical research, social connections to people in power, and exclusive (and exclusionary) ideas about what is legitimate to teach in medical school. Academic pedigree is yet another resource that elite schools have access to and that distinguishes them from "non-elite" schools (I use the term elite because of its place in the sociological canon, whereas the doctors in this book were more tactful: "It is not that [lower-ranked medical school] is nonacademic, it's just that ... you know").

This chapter showcases Eliza, whose attraction to status made her decision to move to the Midwest for her fellowship even more curious. While certainly a reputable program, her fellowship wasn't at an elite research-oriented academic institution. Completing a fellowship there could be viewed as a momentary detour, one she would have to explain (or confess) to her peers. Nonetheless, it was one of the few fellowships that offered the type of specialized surgical training Eliza needed to move toward her long-range goal of improving the health of children in underserved populations. Her story reveals the tension one aspiring doctor felt between stepping off the well-trodden path of elite medicine to do what she needed to do to find meaning versus staying on the narrower path of least resistance that was expected of graduates of elite medical schools.[4]

## "Way leads on to way": The reproduction of elite medicine

In the mid-twentieth century, socialization was often understood as cultural downloading, almost devoid of individuals' capacities to act of their own volition. Since then, understandings have changed, and even the term "socialization" has seemed to fall out of favor.[5] In medical education, socialization has been largely replaced by terms like professionalism, professional identity formation, or the hidden curriculum. However, without socialization, it is easy to lose sight of how people come to know, implicitly if not explicitly, their larger cultural context with its structures, regulations, professional norms, and expectations. I use the term socialization because it accommodates the capacity of longitudinal qualitative studies to trace how individuals are shaped by the culture of medicine and its status hierarchy (that is, a system of social ranking based on relative prestige). In this respect, being socialized into medicine's elite is a reproductive process that preserves hierarchy across generations of doctors. Simply stated, privilege persists. Eliza's story highlights the remarkable power that the culture of medicine and its status hierarchy have in controlling who gets in, who stays in, and who rises to the top.

Medical school is a primary engine for socialization into medicine and its status hierarchy. Some would say that medical schools are where doctors are created. But medical schools as primary engines for socialization are not alike. Seminal work in sociology has proposed that status hierarchies heightened the standing of doctors from certain schools that prioritized research in the biomedical sciences. These doctors generated new, specialized knowledge used to develop clinical practice guidelines for "rank and file" doctors.[6] The former – not the latter – have defined what legitimate knowledge is and what medical students need to know. What distinguishes the research-oriented elite from the rank and file is separate and specialized training, beginning in medical school.[7]

Elite medical schools have a robust research infrastructure necessary to generate new knowledge. Graduates of these schools are expected to be leaders in medicine because they are the ones making exciting discoveries to be used downstream. But what happens when these graduates are not passionate about biomedical research? What if they care more about social science or improving the system that delivers research-informed healthcare?

Medicine is, itself, an elite profession. In that regard, this chapter about being socialized into medicine follows a long line of inquiry about the structure and function of professions. But we know little about how status hierarchy has its effect through the long arc of training.[8] By following a cohort of aspiring doctors from the start of medical school all the way through training and into practice, I watched status hierarchy at work through time by staying with doctors who attended the same elite medical school but ended up in different residencies, different fellowships, and different specialties. In this story of how the academic pedigree that is afforded to those who train at elite medical schools has a lasting impact on their career trajectories, we discover an unexpected outcome. Rather than facilitating career choice, socialization into medicine's elite can unexpectedly narrow the career choices by deeming only some paths worthy of traveling.

## "Looked down as far as I could": The elite medical school path into residency

Getting into medical school is a monumental feat. Years of taking courses to meet the requirements for admission to medical school – a heavy load of biology, chemistry, physics, and math followed by intensive studying for the high-stakes exams – need to be matched with an outstanding grade point average and MCAT score. But superior grades are insufficient. Prospective medical students are encouraged to shadow physicians in healthcare settings, gain experience in research or global health, take on leadership roles, volunteer in hospitals, or even work in some clinical capacity like a medical scribe. Throw in the need to write a compelling personal statement and withstand the pressure of interviews, and it's no wonder that getting into medical school is seen as a significant accomplishment. Acceptance rates at medical schools reflect this highly competitive environment. In 2010, the year this study began, almost 43,000 individuals cleared the hurdles described above and applied to MD-granting medical schools in the United States; of these, a little under half (almost 19,000) enrolled.[9]

Prospective medical students don't just have to brace themselves for four years of unrelenting toil learning the intricacies of medical care. They have to absorb the sticker shock of the cost of medical school. Back in 2010, students were looking at a median four-year cost of attendance at private medical schools in the range of $250,000 (not including living expenses).[10] Suffice it to say that the competition is even stiffer and the price tag even higher for students who want to attend an elite medical school.

It was on the cusp of entering medical school when Eliza first faced the tension that would bubble up time and again as she became a doctor – the attraction of an academic pedigree leading her in one direction, while her medicine-adjacent interest that supported her long-range goal led her in another. On the one hand, there were simple dollars and cents to consider, especially since she had received a scholarship to attend a different medical school that wasn't ranked as elite. But for Eliza, academic pedigree rather than a scholarship was the criterion for success: "I got into a lower-ranked school, which in my head is not as good of a medical school. I decided to pay full tuition and go to an elite school because I just think it's a better school." For many people, taking on substantial student loans when there is an option to emerge from medical school with less debt might be hard to fathom, no matter how elite the alternative is. Eliza could have graduated with less debt, but not without lingering unanswered questions: "I think if I hadn't achieved the success that I had wanted in my career that I would have wondered for the rest of my life if it was because of where I went to medical school ... I didn't want to take any chances."

At the end of her first year in medical school, Eliza assumed that getting accepted had been the hard part. In her mind, everything else was pretty much guaranteed. She got into an elite medical school, and now the doors to opportunity would open:

> I spent a lot of time in college worrying about getting into medical school. But being in this [elite] medical school, I'm not worrying about what am I going to do in the future because you are kind of on this set track already ... It was almost harder to get into medical school than to be in medical school because there was that stress of the uncertainty and wondering if I was going to get in. But now I know that I'm going to get into residency, and now I know I'm going to continue to do something in medicine.

Eliza's assumption wasn't hubris; the statistics bear her out. Nearly all graduates of medical schools in the United States from 2005 to 2015 were admitted into a residency program the same year they graduated.[11] While no exact numbers exist for graduates from elite medical schools, it's even more likely that they were admitted into a residency program. These students have an additional leg up by virtue of their academic pedigree, and as a result, they are more likely to get into the most competitive residencies. But academic pedigree also meant they were channeled along an academic path, with expectations to be leaders in medicine, making discoveries and generating new knowledge. What stands out is the innocuous nature of socialization into the elite pathway. Halfway through her fellowship, Krista recalled,

> I didn't really think a lot about the future steps when I was a medical student. I mean, there was always a focus, at least in my experience as a medical student, on academics as a means to an end, which was residency. I didn't get the sense that they were necessarily trying to funnel us into a strictly academic role, but it was clear they wanted us to match in prestigious programs. And that almost always overlaps with an academic role.

Reflecting on his experience in an elite medical school, Tim actually used the word "inculcated" to describe how these professional norms and expectations had shaped how he thought about his career. He went on to say,

> You were acutely aware and consistently reminded that [elite medical school] is a selective place. It's a place that trains predominately subspecialists with a heavy skew to surgeons. I think coming out of that environment, it still colors the expectations I have of myself. Maybe I would have been more open to other things or at least more exploratory at the outset of my training, rather than being fixated on academic surgery and competitive subspecialty training.

As Tim adroitly said in a later interview, "elite begets elite." Medical students at elite medical schools understood that they needed to do well on standardized tests like the three-part USMLE,[12] get top grades in clerkships, and garner strategic social connections because this combination was their ticket into competitive residencies. At these schools, success meant one thing – moving on to the next prestigious program. In this way, students were socialized to stay on an elite trajectory that narrowed their career options. And shifting away from this trajectory was considered risky, if not downright foolish.

## "Sorry I could not travel both": When interests are at odds

One way that elite medicine narrows career options is its veneration of research in the biomedical sciences and dismissal of other sciences. According to the aspiring doctors in this book, there was a not-so-subtle prejudice against health systems science, where the focus is on system-wide delivery of care, not on discovering new knowledge or translating that knowledge to patient care.[13] This is not to say that health systems science didn't have its advocates. In fact, systems-based practice was recognized by the Accreditation Council of Graduate Medical Education as a core competency domain almost ten years before these doctors entered medical school. But they were taught that anything other than the biomedical sciences was an adjacent interest and not where they should channel most of their time and energy.

Without a doubt, medical education has evolved considerably since 2010, when the doctors in this book were just starting medical school. Today, medical students have to learn to practice in an increasingly complex system of healthcare. Some would argue that health systems science is as foundational to medical education as biomedical science.[14] Nevertheless, the primacy of biomedical science, as the path for the best and the brightest in elite medical schools, is not easily altered.

Of the six doctors in this book, Eliza was one whose long-term goals did not neatly fit into the training provided by elite academic institutions, at least when she started medical school. As she explained, the prevailing stereotype in these institutions was that "pure medicine" simply meant the biomedical sciences:

> The glamorous jobs are like the neurosurgeons of the world – you know, the Nobel Prize winners and the real scientists. In academic medicine, I feel like those are the people with the plaques in the hallways, like this guy won the Nobel Prize, and this guy discovered this molecule, and this guy discovered the treatment for cystic fibrosis. It's all these discoveries – it's the pureness of medicine that is so important here.

Like many medical students, what drew Eliza to medicine was the potential to make a lasting impact in the world. Childhood trips to Southeast Asia stirred in her an interest in providing "high-quality medicine to kids in poorly resourced settings" and became her long-range goal. Initially, she thought that would entail going to other countries to care for individual patients. But her thinking changed at the end of her first year of medical school when she grasped the scope of healthcare disparities that existed locally: "I had this international focus for a long time, and then I came to medical school and realized, 'Oh, there is a lot in the United States that needs to be fixed ... I don't need to look a million miles away.'"

Eliza's sharp analytical mind quickly realized that she could intervene at a systems level, not a individual level: "I realized that one doctor treating a patient one by one is just not efficient. I could grab a backpack and a bunch of medication and go set out and treat people one by one, but that's the least efficient way." From her perspective, she needed to figure out how to improve health systems if she were to achieve her ultimate goal of improving the health of kids in underserved areas.

However, even as a first-year student, Eliza sensed that her interest in health systems was outside the norm of the "science-focused" elite medical school she was attending. She wasn't willing to let go of academic pedigree, but she did pursue extracurricular activities that fed her biomedicine-adjacent interest. She participated in student-run medical clinics for the urban poor, completed a Spanish immersion course in Central America, and helped develop an international health elective for medical students. Eliza debated between pursuing a master's degree in public health (MPH) or a master's degree in business administration (MBA). She chose the latter because, as she put it, "an MBA doesn't overlap at all with medical school. I think that makes it more valuable."

What interested Eliza and what she perceived as an important step toward achieving her long-range goal was perceived as risky by medicine's elite. Eliza knew that having an MBA could send the message that she was not serious about "real medicine":

> I hear different stories of residents who have MBAs being contacted by headhunters and being recruited all the time. Residency programs see that as a risk – if they take an applicant who has an MBA, they may drop out of residency. Or they may get their residency and then go into business and never come back to surgery. It's seen as selling out in the sense that you'll become this person who doesn't treat patients anymore, just makes billions of dollars.

When reflecting on her decision to pursue an MBA, Eliza acknowledged that she was out of step with what was expected of medical students on an elite trajectory. But she was determined to get the training she needed to achieve her goal and make a difference in the world.

Her experience of being out of step was not unique. During her fellowship, Krista pursued a master's degree in a biomedicine-adjacent field and was also warned about the downsides:

> My adviser was like, "It wouldn't hurt to think about getting an MPH because people understand that when they're hiring you; people aren't going to understand this [bioethics] degree." That's hard to hear – that I may not be as desirably employable as if I had different letters after my name, even though this is a robust master's program from a respected institution.

The message was clear to trainees in elite academic institutions: those who veered off the elite trajectory did so at their own risk, jeopardizing (in Eliza's case) the success of their residency applications or (in Krista's case) their job search for attending positions. Staying on an elite trajectory was arduous: long hours of learning on the job and rigorous academic requirements. But it was also the path of least resistance – the path least likely to be challenged by those in charge.

## "Took the other, but just as fair?": The choice of specialization and fitting in

Eliza completed her clerkship rotations, learning firsthand from assisting in patient care and seeing the day-to-day life of doctors. She was surprised to find how much she enjoyed different specialties. Toward the end of her clerkship year, Eliza admitted,

> I loved surgery a lot more than I thought I would – like I didn't think I was going to like it, but it was definitely one of my favorite clerkship rotations ... I don't know what I'm going to end up doing, but it's nice to know that I'll love whatever I do.

Eliza took a gap year during medical school to complete her MBA and to think more about her career. Taking a year off from school to do a master's degree or to do research wasn't exactly the norm, but it was not unusual. For instance, Blake also took a year to complete an MPH.

Eliza was particularly enthusiastic about business school – so much so that there were times when she wondered if her interest in health systems science would outweigh her interest in medicine. But as she reengaged with hands-on patient care during her elective rotations in her final year of medical school, she realized that she would not be satisfied with a career devoid of direct patient contact:

> I'm interested in health systems and how to deliver high-quality healthcare in low-resource settings. I think it's very important, and I definitely like looking at healthcare in the bigger picture. But I also think it's going to be much more fulfilling if I still have those personal connections with patients.

For Eliza, the question was how to fit health systems science into an elite trajectory. This was a Gordian knot that would not be easily cut. The tension was magnified when Eliza felt a strong pull toward surgery. The problem was that surgery wasn't a specialty that could easily accommodate side projects like health systems science. It was a hands-on, skills-based specialty that demanded hours in the operating room, not a highbrow "cerebral specialty": "I was totally surprised that I loved surgery. I thought I was going to like a more cerebral specialty like internal medicine. I liked both but, you know, surgery was – the pace was great for me."

What made her specialty choice even more fraught was that Eliza had not envisioned being a surgeon, unlike some students who, from day one of medical school, pictured themselves as one. For most of medical school, Eliza never doubted her intention to practice medicine in a specialty that could accommodate her interest in health systems science: "I thought the drive to do something compatible with my interests in health systems or the business side of medicine would override my need to do an active specialty where you had more procedures." Even after she made her decision to pursue surgery and applied to residency programs, she second-guessed herself:

> I wish I could say that choosing surgery was a relief, and I just let it go at that moment. But it was terrifying ... When I submitted my residency application, I was like, "Oh my God it's done, I'm so happy." For a few days I was like, "Yes, I'm done, it's over, and now it's out of my hands." But then, of course, the doubts start creeping in, and I started wondering, "Did I make the right choice?" And then there were moments when I was like, "This is the wrong choice. Oh my God, how do I get myself out of this? Do I really want to be a surgeon?"

Eliza wasn't alone in feeling uncertain about her specialty choice; everyone in this book grappled with this decision to some degree. But the questions that plagued Eliza were unnerving because they pointed to the Gordian knot. On the one hand, Eliza adored surgery. "There is part of me that super-loves it." She especially loved that it was matter of fact and found it fulfilling when she was able to fix things. But on the other hand, she recognized that surgery could pull her away from health systems science:

> I was scared about becoming a surgeon, not because you have to do surgery, but because you have to be a surgeon.

That basically takes away a lot of what matters to me. If I was an emergency medicine doctor, I could work shifts. But if you're a surgeon, you have to be a surgeon a lot of the time – it's like no sleep, no food, just do surgery. I'm not really like that, and so that's scary to me. Surgery definitely funnels you.

To Eliza, it felt like an impossible choice. If she chose surgery, she'd have to sacrifice her passion for health systems science and potentially her long-range goal. But if she didn't choose surgery, she would not be happy in her day-to-day work. When she was nearing the end of her second year in residency, she framed her dilemma like this:

My biggest fear is that I'll come out of residency and have no purpose. I only became a surgeon because I loved the actual hands-on thing so much. I fought that decision for a long time. I was so upset that that was what my body and brain were moving me to, because I don't really want to be a surgeon. I don't feel like a stereotypical surgeon.

Eliza made it clear that she was not the *"Grey's Anatomy* type: all in, no sleep, no food, just do surgery." She was drawn to – and intentional about – working with underserved populations. Had she not had an interest in health systems science, she could settle for being "just a surgeon." But it wasn't that simple:

Part of me wishes I could have just become a surgeon. I totally see the appeal of that, but I would hate myself if I did. I get scared because my interests are so far apart from each other that I am going to come out of this in the middle – which is nothing.

## "Telling with a sigh": The pressures and pulls of residency

Eliza's fear was that surgery would frustrate her pursuit of health systems science was not off the mark. She matched to a competitive residency program at an academic medical center, which satisfied her attraction to reputation and name recognition and afforded her plenty of time to do surgery. But residency amounted to a constant pressure to focus solely on surgery, leaving little room for any outside interests. Eliza was expected to work hard and learn on the job, hour after hour after hour. It proved to be a strange combination: "I love it and hate it at the same time." Midway through residency, she listed things that she learned so far. One was learning the skills of her surgical subspecialty. Another was learning what kind of person she was under pressure. A third was learning how much she didn't know. And last was learning how much she loved the complex mechanics of surgery:

> When surgery is involved, you're cutting into a patient and doing harm before you do good – always. But the thing is, I love it. I'm very happy with what I am doing. The interventions themselves are very involved and can be morbid, so it's confusing sometimes. But the thing is, I surprisingly get so much joy from actually doing the intervention, from literally the physical act of doing surgery.

Reflecting back on her specialty choice, Eliza acknowledged that other specialties might have better accommodated her interest in health systems science, but she would have missed out on something she loved. Early in residency, she remarked that she had "dodged a bullet" by choosing surgery over a medical specialty. But it wasn't all roses. Surgical residency lost some luster as it dragged on. Eliza was operating almost every day and spending long hours in outpatient clinics. Part of what made residency so arduous for Eliza was that the day-to-day grind prohibited time to engage in anything other than surgery. When she was in medical school, she could legitimately devote time to health systems science by pursuing an MBA. But there was no time for health systems science in residency. It was designed to prepare her for surgical practice – no more and nothing less. In fact, given that health systems science was a second-class citizen compared to biomedical science, Eliza had to censor her interest to avoid being pegged as (in her words) "a traitor." She went on to share this:

> I have an attending who I really, really respect, and every time we have a meeting and talk about quality metrics, which are really important for systems improvement, he just rolls his eyes and says, "Why are they telling us what to do? I know what to do." But to me, it's just really interesting. I feel almost like the enemy, like I'm in stealth mode. I have to joke a lot, like, "Ha ha, this is stupid," that kind of thing.

Eliza recognized the lack of support for her interests in health systems science as unfair. Residency was five years of her life, and it felt wrong to ask her to put her interests on hold when the same was not asked of other residents. Why did she have to feel like "the enemy" when she pursued her interests, but others did not?

> I think it's unfair to not be able to pursue your other interests. I mean, five years is a long time. Some people choose to have kids when they are in residency, and everyone applauds them for taking time to pursue those interests. But somehow if you're interested in health systems, they're like, "You should be focusing on surgery." It's frowned upon; it's ridiculed. You're supposed to hide those things.

In line with her characteristic persistence, Eliza's perception of this unfairness did not lead to outright resignation on her part. She managed to find ways to nurture her interest in health systems science by joining the hospital's committee to address patient safety and quality healthcare. But when it came to more active engagement in health systems science, Eliza acknowledged, "I'm still interested, but I keep trying to remember that I'm in training. I can't do all the things I want to do in residency." On the cusp of fellowship, Eliza decided that her drive to do health systems science would need to be temporarily muted, though not totally silenced. She would focus on the nuts and bolts of surgery during her fellowship and her first year of being an attending: "I'm really trying to focus on becoming the best surgeon, learning the most, and then figuring out what that's going to look like for wherever I end up."

## "The road less traveled": A surprising fellowship

Eliza was in residency at the same academic institution for five years, so it wasn't until she explored subspecialty training via fellowships that the lure of academic pedigree again came to the fore. She could pursue any number of fellowships and subspecialize in different areas, some more prestigious and lucrative than others. As she explored her options, she realized that if she opted for a fellowship program affiliated with an elite medical school, she would likely sacrifice learning to do the types of surgeries she really wanted to do – ones that were less glamorous but spoke to her long-term goal to improve the health of children in underserved populations. Conversely, if she opted to do a fellowship outside an elite institution, she'd veer off the elite trajectory, and there would be an anomaly in her academic pedigree. Should she do a fellowship with a name school or a fellowship that would better accommodate her interests? Eliza's struggle to choose a fellowship program shows just how tenacious the professional norms and expectations of graduates of elite medical schools can be:

> When I was applying to fellowship, I was embarrassed to say that I really wanted to go to a program in the Midwest. Initially I almost didn't rank it [highly]. I almost put [several elite institutions] above it, even though for me, they weren't the right fit ... I was like, how can I get away from being at an elite school?

In the end, Eliza chose the fellowship program in the Midwest, the one that could readily accommodate her surgical interests. She opted out of a fellowship program at an elite academic institution. Did she have some regrets? Perhaps. Her choice was the source of some "embarrassment": "The fellowship I did was, externally, not as prestigious as places like Harvard or Stanford. Those are names [that] didn't really mean anything, but they were names that I liked to hear." Nonetheless, the tradeoff seemed to work in her favor. At the end of her fellowship, Eliza reported,

> I LOVED fellowship. There so many moments of learning, both peaks and valleys. As a fellow, you have a different relationship with residents below you and all of a sudden, you're learning how to teach in the OR, how to not do everything yourself and allow for mistakes to happen that you'll have to fix. Really, you're imagining yourself as an attending.

Fellowship turned out to be more than learning how to do specialized surgeries and learning how to teach. Eliza found herself supported by a female mentor who encouraged her to be herself and "just do you." Up to this point, she had often tried to live her life according to what was expected of her as a graduate of an elite medical school. Now she was giving herself the green light to not do that: "To have women who have been through it, who are successful surgeons, and who did it their own way ... that encourages me to do my own thing. That's really valuable and something I've been missing."

## Conclusion: "Keeping the first for another day"?

After four years in medical school plus a gap year, five years in residency, and one year in fellowship, Eliza was finally an attending in surgery. Although she was offered jobs in private hospitals, she opted for a job at the same place where she did her residency. On top of establishing a surgical practice and supervising residents and fellows, she started building programs within her department, which allowed her to dip her toe in health systems science. Her training, her experience with hospital committees, and her MBA prepared her for a role with more depth than surgical responsibilities alone. Eliza routinely spoke of being "more than just a surgeon":

> Sometimes I wonder if I should have done more to focus. But I have a lot of different interests, and I want more than just being a surgeon. The health systems science stuff is SO interesting ... Doing surgery is hard, but that's really just kind of being a mechanic or an artisan. You're just using your hands, and that is almost the fun part. I feel like my real work will be trying to figure out how to make these changes in the health systems in underserved communities that I care about.

In Eliza's story, surgery was in tension with health systems science which, in turn, was in tension with the expectations of graduates of elite medical schools. After her fellowship ended, Eliza admitted that she hadn't totally let go of that attraction to reputation and name recognition:

"There's this lingering expectation that you will go into academia and be a doctor at an elite medical school. I've not been able to let go of that; it's hard for me to think about not being in a place with all kinds of resources." But her metrics for grading success were in flux. As a newly minted attending, she was seeing that, from a hospital perspective, success was how much money she could bring in. From an elite medical school perspective, success was how much research she could get funded. But Eliza didn't want either of those to define her success. She couldn't take away the name of the elite medical school she attended or the professional norms and expectations that came with that name. But she could follow the advice given to her as a fellow: to do her own thing. Eliza stayed in academic medicine yet charted her own path. She acknowledged the awkward pull to academic pedigree without losing sight of her long-range goal to do something that mattered. Hers was the road less traveled among the elite in medicine. Staying on that road was her real work.

CHAPTER 2

# Alan's Story About Agency

Let me but do my work from day to day,
In field or forest, at the desk or loom,
In roaring market-place or tranquil room;
Let me but find it in my heart to say,
When vagrant wishes beckon me astray,
"This is my work; my blessing, not my doom;
Of all who live, I am the one by whom
This work can best be done in the right way."

Then shall I see it not too great, nor small,
To suit my spirit and to prove my powers;
Then shall I cheerful greet the labouring hours,
And cheerful turn, when the long shadows fall
At eventide, to play and love and rest,
Because I know for me my work is best.
– Henry van Dyke, "Work"

## Introduction: "Let me but do my work from day to day"

On the sixth ring, Alan picked up his phone. He said a quick hello and apologized for the delay in answering: "I was on call last night but wanted to spend a little time in my shop before calling it a day." Even though Alan worked in a procedure-rich field in medicine that demanded skillful use of his hands, he still unwound after a long shift by using them more.

The work that drew him to his shop was far from patient care. It was marquetry, a decorative technique where wood veneers are sawed into shapes and then assembled into intricate patterns, not unlike a stained-glass window. Alan was eager to tell me about his latest piece, a side table for his living room. His description was exacting in its level of detail – the type of wood, the application of the lacquer, even the order of the steps he took when assembling the piece – nothing was left to chance.

Alan had always been drawn to the arts; in fact, he had a career in music prior to entering medicine. His passion for all things artistic was also evident in medical school. In his last year, he completed an independent art elective. For Alan, art wasn't just a creative outlet. As an aspiring doctor, it altered the way he viewed patients clinically and gave him a vantage point from which he could better see the human dimension of their medical issues. He recalled the marquetry piece he did in his art elective that portrayed the devastation that comes with suddenly learning that one has a life-changing illness:

> I spent the whole month on a picture to represent a compelling case that I saw in the emergency room. This woman came in

with a zoster infection, a pretty standard case. She was in a lot of pain and had the classic localized dermatome rash. I went in, talked to her, did an exam, and noticed that she had a diffuse rash all over. I looked it up and it turned out that it could be a sign of HIV. When I asked her about HIV, she didn't know anything about it. We did a test, and … she ended up positive.

What made this case stand out was Alan's realization that doctors were not detached characters in stories of pivotal moments. Doctors bore witness to those moments where patients' lives could change in an instant:

For me, it was this moment of clarity when you realize that coming into the hospital can be a life-changing event. For this woman, finding out that you have this little infection seems pretty normal, but then finding out that you have this illness that's never going to go away and may actually kill you – that can be devastating.

Some of Alan's classmates had gone into medicine because they saw it as a lucrative career, and one that promised public respect and recognition. But moments of clarity like the one Alan described above helped him recognize that he was not drawn to money or recognition. What he wanted was to make a demonstrable difference in patients' lives. Not surprisingly, Alan was drawn to the acute-care surgical fields where every patient encounter was pivotal: "Somebody comes in for surgery because they really need it … they're going to die without it, or they're in pain or they've lost function and you're trying to fix that. Every patient encounter is a life-changing encounter."

For Alan, using his hands was just as important as making a difference in patients' lives. This showed up in his art as well as his work. He hadn't always felt that the importance of what he did would be based on his personal values. Earlier in life, he aspired to "do something big" – something others attributed value to. "Growing up, my aspirations as a kid were to be some kind of rock star, something a little out of reality." That aspiration to "do something big" was confirmed when he was admitted to an elite medical school. Just like how in Eliza's story we saw that elite medical schools had high expectations of students, Alan recalled, "It's like there was a little voice in the back of my mind saying, 'You got into an elite medical school – the world is your oyster. You should do something big.'"

But Alan's thinking changed over the four years of medical school. The test of Alan's position about appraising his work for how it fit with his life and his values came when he had to choose a specialty. Much like how art altered the way he thought of patients so that he could see their humanness, art also altered the way he looked at his career:

> I know the purpose of these arts-in-medicine courses is to look at patients from a different angle, to see where they're coming from and understand them on a deeper level. But you can take that same process and look at yourself to find out, instead of what treatment do you need, what career path do you need, what can you live with, and what's important to you.

Alan realized that a meaningful career in medicine wasn't necessarily "doing something big": going for the money, respect, prestige, and admiration. He needed work that would align with his values and make sense for the rest of his life. So he shifted away from thinking about a career that thrived solely on acute, life-changing consequences to thinking about a career that would allow him to experience those high-adrenaline moments but not at the exclusion of living a life outside of the operating room:

> I liked surgery, don't get me wrong. And it is a career that's presented as big in elite medical schools. If I didn't have to live the surgeon's life, surgery would have been great. I would have really enjoyed surgery because I really like doing procedures. But the other things surgeons must do would have made me miserable.

Alan had moved on from his first career in music because it wasn't sustainable as a lifestyle. And ultimately that's also what drove his decision to pursue anesthesia.

## "Let me but find it in my heart to say": The temporality of agency

Alan's capacity to choose what he valued *and* what he could live with is an expression of *agency*. It sounds deceptively simple. Yet the concept of agency is elusive, and its understanding is muddled. In their seminal article, "What Is Agency?," sociologists Mustafa Emirbayer and Ann Mische list terms that are associated with agency: selfhood, motivation, will, purposiveness, intentionality, choice, initiative, freedom, and creativity.[1] Medical educators would probably include terms like self-direction and autonomy. What Emirbayer and Mische add to the agency literature is a temporal dimension. They claim that to really understand agency, it must be situated in the flow of time. To that end, they conceptualize agency as a temporally embedded process of social engagement. It's dynamic inner work, shaped by the past but also oriented toward the future while residing in the present. Agency has a past: preceding events, triggers, and moments of clarity like the one Alan described when he realized that encounters with doctors can be life-changing. Agency also has a future: a capacity to imagine different possibilities like Alan did when he toggled between "doing something big" or doing something he could live with. And agency has a present: making decisions when the "rubber meets the road." There was, for instance, a point in time when Alan had to be pragmatic and decide which specialty to pursue.

As we learned from Eliza, status hierarchies in medicine can narrow the choice of medical specialties students consider, making it appear as if their options are limited. Her story provides a contrast to Alan, where agency helps to explain his career choice. What I found in the stories of these medical trainees was that moments where they made career decisions – e.g., medical students choosing a specialty or residents choosing where to practice after graduation – were the most vivid pictures of agency as a temporally embedded process, informed by the past, enacted in the present, and oriented toward the future. But because medical educators have typically conceptualized agency as self-direction or autonomy in context-specific, time-limited, cross-sectional studies that ask trainees to remember back or speculate about their future, there is much we don't know about the temporal dimension of agency that longitudinal explorations could reveal.

To complicate matters further, the exercise of agency does not manifest itself in exactly the same way in an individual over time. As Emirbayer and Mische explain, individuals expressing agency are simultaneously oriented toward the past, present, and future; "they switch between (or 'recompose') their temporal orientations."[2] People constantly shift between different time perspectives as they make decisions, allowing them to creatively navigate and make conscious choices within the limitations and opportunities presented by their circumstances. Sometimes the past weighs more heavily for one decision (e.g., the decision whether or not to get remarried), whereas in other instances the future might exert more of a hold on an individual's decision (e.g., one's willingness to take an experimental drug when faced with a life-limiting diagnosis). In sum, individuals engage in the temporally embedded process of agency differently depending on their unique past, present, and future – the frame of which is constantly changing as they live their lives and acquire new experiences and new ideas.

What Alan's story highlights, in addition to agency's temporal dimension, is something often lost in theoretical discussions of agency: choosing *not* to do something. While it's a well-known platitude that every decision is a choice, his experiences reveal the importance attached to agency with respect to being able to say no. While trainees and even junior faculty are often advised to say yes to every opportunity that comes their way, Alan's story reveals how agency is reflected just as much in the opportunities we say no to as the opportunities we say yes to. To be clear, as a white male – the majority group in academic medicine – Alan could say no to things that minority group members could not.[3] Nevertheless, his story reveals how careful consideration of his options led him to opt out of things typically expected of elite medical school graduates when they did not make sense for how he envisioned his life and what he valued.

## "In field or forest, at the desk or loom": The whole picture when applying to medical school

In the search for characteristics that make a good doctor, medical schools seek a diverse applicant pool, and ultimately a diverse student body. To those ends, schools are adopting holistic reviews of prospective students, which consider not only academic metrics but also attributes and experiences that might not connect directly to medicine. Since the application process is highly competitive, the question then arises: what "holistic" experiences and characteristics do medical schools look for?

The answer is not so clear. According to the Association of American Medical Colleges, holistic review is an admissions process that considers each applicant individually by balancing their academic profile with personal experiences and attributes.[4] Admission committee members understand that the path to medical school may not be smooth or linear, and from a holistic perspective they focus instead on how life experiences are integrated and what lessons are learned. For example, special consideration might be given to applicants whose stories show significant growth and outstanding character, particularly in the face of adversity. In addition to applicant characteristics, holistic review also considers how well each applicant's aspirations align with the mission of the medical school. Thus, the nature of holistic review varies across schools.

If the goal of medical schools is to recruit a diverse student body, then Alan should have been at the top of any medical school's list. He started medical school when he was in his early thirties with a decade of life experiences already in the rearview mirror. Alan studied music education in college, but after realizing that teaching wasn't for him, he switched to music performance. He tried his hand working as an itinerant musician, teaching piano lessons to supplement his income, but basically living out of his car between gigs as a jazz pianist. This left him with plenty of time on his hands to think about his future. He particularly enjoyed popular science books and even toyed with the idea of pursuing astronomy. But, in his mind, medicine was a science that offered a lot of different options. "You could do hard science. You can do clinical work; you can do procedures. You can do outpatient, inpatient medicine, you know, all kinds of ways that you could do it." It was the diversity of options in medicine that sealed his decision to go to medical school.

So Alan changed course and pursued a career in medicine. To be a viable candidate for medical school, he had to build his academic profile almost from scratch. He did well on the MCAT and took night classes to complete prerequisite courses. During the day, he worked in the IT Department for a brokerage company and, through on-the-job training, learned the basics of software engineering. Unbeknownst to Alan at the time, those skills would prove to be quite profitable down the road.

Alan's academic profile was solid but did not distinguish him from the other applicants. In a time of holistic admissions, students need to stand out from the crowd. In this respect, what others might see as a failed career as a pianist was an asset. He suspected that he benefited from his atypical past because it caught the eye of the admissions dean:

> My GPA and my MCAT score were good but average for [elite schools]. I didn't get that many interviews for medical school because I was a risky candidate. Honestly, I think what got me in was that the Dean of the Admissions Committee had also been a pianist. And if she hadn't been on the committee, I'm not sure I would have gotten in.

While there are no "golden tickets" for medical school admission, Alan's musical background was something that set him apart from his classmates and enhanced (on some level) the diversity of the student body. But his life experience did much more than diversify. Viewing agency as a temporal process, we can see that his past became a well that he drew from in a variety of unexpected ways when making career decisions moving forward.

## "When vagrant wishes beckon me astray": Dispositions veil and hierarchy constrains agency

Getting into medical school is an act of differentiation – setting yourself apart from the crowd so that the admissions committee notices you. But being in medical school is an act of assimilation. The discourse of diversity that emphasizes individuality and difference among medical school applicants is replaced by the discourse of standardization that strives for homogeneity and sameness. It might be surprising, then, to learn that in medical school, the expectation to "take initiative" was a favored and more or less standardized disposition.[5]

Initiative might seem like agency in the way students "put themselves out there" (in the words of Alan). But taking initiative wasn't about being different or pursuing one's interests – it was a common attitude that students learned to adopt and embrace because that was what all "high-flying" medical students did. In other words, "taking initiative" was what they were *expected* to do in order to succeed in an elite medical school. It was "taking the initiative" in name only.

Alan was no different. Early in his first year, he was already rattling off the numerous things he did in extracurricular clubs. One of those clubs introduced medical students to careers in surgery and promoted interactions among medical students and surgeons:

> We signed up [to be on transplant call], and then they assigned us times. I got the pager one week and got called up. I know a fair number of people have gone on transplant call. I might be the only one that saw trauma surgery. All of this is new to me, so I get excited about this stuff pretty easily.

While "taking initiative" had an appearance of agency in medical school, the hierarchy in healthcare openly constrained agency. Medical students were encouraged to see themselves as integral members of the healthcare team. But even before they were exposed to the full complement of how hierarchy manifests, from the physician-in-chief all the way down to the food service workers, students were acutely aware that they would need to navigate the "layers." As Krista said, "We're used to deferring to authority, so it will be interesting to see how we maintain our sense of not thinking, 'I'm just the little gopher medical student, I know nothing.' Because really, we essentially know nothing."

It wasn't until much later in training that the doctors in this book talked about feeling like important team members. As medical students, they were thrilled when they were allowed to actively engage in some of the real work of a doctor, even if the work had minimal significance. Alan described these instances as "a little taste of the goal" – a peek at his future self. What he could not fully appreciate was that what was thrilling to him as a medical student would become extraordinarily mundane as a resident.

## "To suit my spirit and to prove my powers": The sub-internship

In the last two years of medical school, Alan faced a crucial choice about the specialty he would pursue and thus the kind of doctor he'd become. Halfway through his clerkship year, he was convinced that he was drawn to acute care and surgery:

> Being in the emergency room and holding pressure on the knife wounds of a patient, it all reaffirms what I've come to realize over these six months – I'm going to want to go into something hands-on, where I'm physically doing something rather than managing someone's medication or dealing with them psychologically.

What is more, Alan was drawn to a career that would accommodate "using my hands" – hints of the former jazz pianist in him peeking through. From his perspective, a meaningful career would be one that fit these pieces together. His initial inclination – rooted in both his childhood aspiration to be a rock star and the expectations of students in elite medical schools – was to chase his grandest ambitions:

> My initial instinct was ... what's the *biggest* way I can be in medicine? You know, what's the most exciting thing I can do in medicine? What's the thing in medicine that's going to get me the most attention?

Nevertheless, when Alan looked back at his path to medical school and tried to imagine his future, the question he found himself asking was not, "What's the biggest way I can be in medicine?" Rather, the question was, "Where am I going to put the limit on ambition?" He recognized that "doing something big" would take him down a very different path in medicine than finding a job he'd enjoy doing every day for twenty years. The trick was finding that job.

He was exposed to specialties like internal medicine, primary care, and surgery in his clerkship year, but not others. And if he didn't learn about other specialties, they weren't a viable career path. It was a sub-internship that afforded Alan exposure to anesthesiology. In the United States, a sub-internship is an elective clinical rotation in a student's fourth year of medical school. They are completed within a specialty of interest, typically over the course of a month. Even more than students in clerkships, students in sub-internships gain a sense of responsibility for patient care while still being closely supervised. These experiences, along with feedback from medical school faculty upon completion, let students gauge the specialty's fit.

Alan was settled on using his hands, but there were still many options – first and foremost surgery. But seeing what was expected of surgeons, both in training and later in practice, gave Alan pause.

> If I didn't have to live the surgeon's life, surgery would have been a great thing. I really like doing procedures. But the length of training and the other things they have to do were just too much and would have made me miserable. And I don't think I would have thrived in a surgery residency, not

to mention the impact of being an older married person with little kids as a surgery resident.

Surgical training demanded an unenviable amount of time and effort. But choosing anesthesia meant he had to grapple with the stereotype that anesthesia was a cop-out for students who can't handle surgery. Alan asked himself, "Am I limiting myself by going into anesthesia? Am I cutting off the ability to do something great?" As it turned out, what other students might have seen as a cop-out proved to be a selling point for Alan. Being a surgeon would not offer him the work-life balance he sought after spending his twenties effectively on call every night playing piano. And as a relative latecomer to the field of medicine, he had fewer years in which to pay off his loans and achieve a comfortable nest egg for his family. In other words, surgery would be exciting and get him attention, but it wouldn't fit with the life he envisioned for himself:

> It's figuring out all of this – not just how much money do I need to make, how much time do I need to have off, but even little things like "Am I a morning person? Am I a night person? Do I like talking to people? Do I prefer to only interact with other doctors? Do I like to write? Do I like to read? Do I like to use my hands? Do I like to sit in the dark? Can I stand in the OR for hours?"

Factoring in all the answers to those questions, Alan became convinced that he wanted to specialize in anesthesia – to the point that when his anesthesia sub-internship was over, he found himself asking, "Why do I have to move on? Can't I just stay here?" The more time he spent doing anesthesia and talking to anesthesiologists, the more "everything just kind of clicked." It was the combination of seeing his past, present, and future self reflected in the field of anesthesia that made it "a perfect fit."

## "This is my work; my blessing, not my doom": Narrowing one's focus

Choosing a specialty is one thing; choosing where to do a residency is another. The word "choosing" is somewhat of a misnomer. The National Residency Matching Program is an independent organization that uses a mathematical algorithm to place applicants into residency programs.[6] This algorithm is intended to create a more even playing field.

However, by virtue of attending an elite medical school, the doctors in this book were well-positioned to match into the residency programs they wanted. Some residencies are more academically oriented while others cater to clinical practice. And, as we saw with Eliza, graduates of elite medical schools were channeled into research-intensive academic residencies.

Alan tipped his hand toward his future career path when he highly ranked anesthesia residency programs that were oriented toward clinical practice, not research. Although there were no guarantees, his rankings made it clear that he prioritized programs that would cater to his clinical proclivity:

> They told me, "If you want to stay here [at the elite medical school] for residency, we are almost definitely going to take you in the anesthesia program. You just rank us high, and we will take you." But it was an academic residency. Almost everyone went on to do a fellowship and to do research. It was expected that if you went there for residency, you were going down that academic medicine track. And I didn't think that was going to be for me … so I sculpted my residency toward private practice.

Alan's language of "sculpting" his residency was another manifestation of agency at work – saying no to "going big" in medicine, no to surgery, and no to a research-oriented, academic residency. He was instead saying yes to a career in medicine that best fit *his* life and values.

Alan's first year of a four-year residency (also called an internship) entailed rotating, one month at a time, through different specialties. On paper, internship is when he would gain the prerequisite knowledge and skills he would need for more anesthesia-focused training in the subsequent three years. But in reality, internship was twelve months of doing a lot of nonclinical administrative tasks affectionally known as "scutwork":

> The work, especially as an intern, is almost all junk. It's like calling in scripts to pharmacies, getting in touch with social workers to get someone transportation to go home, or having to explain to a patient why I am not giving them the prescription for pain meds that they want – stuff like that.

Alan's experiences with scutwork as an intern weren't all for naught because, if anything, they confirmed his career choice. For example, he spent time caring for outpatients in clinics, which heightened his desire to work in a surgical setting instead. This was important information for career decision-making because saying no to one option was as important as saying yes to another. Years later, Alan would give similar advice to medical students:

> Students always want to know, "How did you decide what specialty to go into?" I always tell them that one of the most important things they will learn is what they *don't* like. That's even more important than what they do like ... I knew that I liked procedures and the operating room. But that was in part because I knew that I didn't like clinics or sitting in front of computers. I knew the type of work that didn't interest me.

Alan was not unique among the aspiring doctors in this book: all of them expressed a sense of confirmation when they were immersed in their chosen specialty. However, Alan was the one who knew better than anyone, perhaps because of his prior life experience, that excitement can fade. So it was important to know that the work is important even if it doesn't always feel that way:

> I'm getting really good at intubating people, monitoring blood pressure and heart rate. But then I'm charting, filling out forms, plugging in numbers. These are important even if they're not at all enjoyable ... And so, yeah, the work is

important. But I would add that *knowing* that the work is important is also really important because that is what gets you through the tough times.

## "I am the one by whom / This work can best be done": The choices residents face

Anesthesiology training began in earnest in Alan's second year of residency. No longer an intern, he assumed the role of a junior anesthesia resident and started working in the operating room under the supervision of attendings who were credentialed anesthesiologists. His rotations built on each other, starting with easier ones. As a junior resident, Alan took on straightforward cases compared to the ones he would take on as a senior resident – patients who were not as sick, conditions that were not as life-threatening, and risks that were not as high. With each rotation, he gained confidence in doing these bread-and-butter cases, with the ever-present knowledge that even in these cases, anesthesia could kill someone if not done properly:

> You can think of anesthesia as putting someone in a life-threatening situation. It's like a controlled fire that you might set to stop a bigger forest fire. You're stopping people from breathing, you're stopping their heart from doing its job properly, you are putting them at risk for all kinds of complications in order to be able to do surgery. If you are not on top of it and able to deal with those problems, then you have really serious outcomes.

Bread-and-butter cases were the foundational for learning to be an anesthesiologist, but complications took these cases to the next level. What made the operating room a challenging place to learn about complications, compared to other clinical settings, was that anesthesia residents couldn't take a break to strategize. They knew that an attending was supervising and could deal with complications, but there was still a very low margin for error. A big part of progressing in anesthesia residency was starting to learn what to do when things went wrong. And with that progression was a shift in responsibility: "More and more now I'm the one who is going to be expected to take care of these patients when things go wrong."

In addition to dealing with complications, Alan started to care for sicker patients. For example, in his third year of residency, he found himself on a relatively dull post-anesthesia care rotation. Most of the time, he was dealing with routine post-operative issues like pain, nausea, and blood pressure instability. But the rotation came with a wild card – residents were also carrying the code bag. They were the ones who would be called for an emergency intubation – when a patient on one of the regular hospital floors was having a heart attack or was in severe respiratory distress. Typically, residents would wait for their attending and then intubate with them present. But when a patient was actively dying, the resident had to act on their own. As Alan put it,

> If someone is having a code, they [other doctors on regular hospital floors] are doing chest compressions, and the patient is actively dying, so you just go and do it. You don't

wait for your attending; you don't wait for anybody else. You are the anesthesiologist there. That is a big thing … It's your airway. It's your intubation. You're the one making all the decisions.

Alan's comments about making all the decisions point to autonomy in medical training. Much like how "taking initiative" looked like agency in medical school (but perhaps was not), autonomy in residency could be conceptualized as a form of bounded agency, that is, exercising agency within a particular context.[7] Alan had the freedom to make some choices, even if he was a trainee. But unlike agency, someone external to Alan still had to grant autonomy. His attendings and residency program leadership entrusted him with the care of critically ill patients, and that included the freedom to make some choices about patient care. In a similar vein, Krista shared contexts in which she was given the freedom to make choices when she was a senior resident: "I was given a lot of autonomy for some of the general pediatric patients, like how to lead the team, when and how to provide education on rounds, and guiding decision-making on rounds." They didn't quite have agency – the capacity to act completely on their own – yet. It wasn't until after training that Alan was able to make decisions without being granted autonomy by someone else. He described the transition to unsupervised practice like this:

> You have to break the feeling of, "Oh, here's my idea; here's what I want to do, but I'd better run it by somebody." Instead of that you say, "This is what I'm going to do. I'm going to

deal with the consequences if there are any. I'm going to take complete ownership of this decision."

## "Not too great, nor small": Saying no to fellowship, yes to private practice

Midway through residency, Alan made another crucial career decision in choosing to be a generalist rather than do a fellowship in something like cardiac anesthesia or pediatric anesthesia:

> I'm planning NOT to do a fellowship. I'm just going to do general anesthesia. Honestly, I don't need to be at the cutting edge, doing the biggest surgeries, the most exciting surgeries. I'm actually happy doing more general stuff, more fundamental anesthesia.

Eliza's chapter delved into the expectations that graduates of elite medical schools will lead the field by making exciting new discoveries and generating knowledge via biomedical research that would be used downstream by doctors in the "rank and file." By choosing not to do a fellowship, Alan was again saying no to the expected path. Reflecting back on his last year of residency, Alan admitted that his decision to forgo fellowship may have surprised his younger self. However, it made sense given the demands and contingencies of his present:

> I think I would have been surprised about not doing a fellowship if you told me so five years ago when I was a medical

student. But it doesn't surprise me now. Back then, maybe I would have more ambition to do bigger and more exciting things. But now, I don't know ... it kind of feels right. I'm getting older, starting a family. I'm ready to move on.

Once his residency ended, Alan hit the ground running in his first year of practice as an attending anesthesiologist: a new city, a new state, a new set of colleagues, and a new private practice group. He was essentially a private contractor with privileges at a large hospital and its surgical centers. Joining a new practice group, he found himself vaulted from his lower standing as a trainee to being on equal footing with his partners, who were also attending anesthesiologists. While his coresidents who stayed in research-oriented academic institutions would be starting at the bottom, taking the cases that those with seniority did not want, Alan started near the top. He didn't have the luxury of working up to more difficult cases. He also expected to be at a lower tier of knowledge and skills compared to his partners because they had more experience. Instead, he found himself at ease with the technical and clinical aspects of anesthesiology. Gone were the days when life-threatening events were new and exciting. Now these events happened regularly. What had thrown Alan out of his comfort zone as a resident was now a chance to step in and get something done: "You know how to do it right, so you just make it happen." As we will learn in Tim's chapter, achieving that degree of comfort took years of training.

Thus, Alan began his career as a founding partner at a large hospital doing high-acuity cases. It was sink or swim – and Alan thrived:

You never know how you're going to perform until you're the last person in line with no supervision, until you're completely on your own, with no net. "Is my training adequate? Has somebody been propping me up this entire time, and I have just been doing okay? Or do I actually have the skills to do what I need to do?" I've been working without a net this year, and I've had no problems so far.

As time passed, Alan talked about "just working," which meant keeping up his skills and doing his job well but not engaging in any more formal training. He was done with that. He also found himself doing basic procedures like nerve blocks over and over again. But because these procedures offered patients for whom he was responsible some welcome relief from unbearable pain, they didn't seem mundane in the same way that scutwork seemed as a resident. Alan made this comparison:

We see a lot of motor vehicle accidents, patients with broken ribs that hurt like heck. They call us, and we come in and do a nerve block. All of a sudden, their pain goes away; they can breathe. It feels good to do that. Even though the procedure itself is routine and there's scutwork to it like writing orders, it's still very satisfying.

It was on the management side of private practice that Alan began to feel constrained. The infrastructure of most private practice groups is set up to help anesthesiologists focus on patient care and clinical duties rather than get weighed down by the demands of business and financial management. Nonetheless, in joining a new private practice group, Alan was thrust into management, even though he confessed, "I've never been interested in the business side of things." Interest aside, taking on management roles was a way for him to establish himself, and so he took the lead in determining how operating rooms were staffed. To his credit, Alan adroitly married his day job with his software engineering skills garnered in his premedical school days by creating a scheduling program to facilitate the task of staffing operating rooms:

> When I got into practice, our scheduling program – well, it wasn't even a program, it was a Word document. So to fix that, I wrote a little program for doing our room assignments. And that program exploded into our employee portal, and now all our scheduling is done with software that I've written.

Over the course of several years, Alan's managerial work started to overshadow his clinical work. To date, he had dutifully said yes to management, and he certainly wasn't alone in doing so. Eliza shared something similar: "At the beginning of my practice, I have to say yes to everything and every person that comes along and then see where that takes me. I can't be picky." But by now, Alan reached the tipping point: "I don't really want to be in this much management. I would much rather be clinical. I'm just surprised that I do as much management as I do." Things came to a head when he was asked to take over as director of operations; a promotion to be sure, but not the chance to shed managerial roles and tap his creative nature. Consistent with previous times when he had said no to doing something big in medicine, Alan said no to the promotion: "What I really want to do is make stuff. So I opted out. I think it was the right choice. I can't just say yes to everything." Instead, he set out on a career venture, staying with the clinical side of his job but also taking the scheduling software program he had developed for the practice and trying to commercialize it.

## Conclusion: "I know for me my work is best"

What we see in Alan's story is agency as a process that is embedded in the past, present, and future. More than the other doctors in this book, Alan said no to things expected of graduates of elite medical schools, which turned out to be the boldest form of agency. To be clear, all of the aspiring doctors reflected on the choices that got them to where they were a decade after starting medical school. And they were, by and large, content with their choices, whether or not that entailed saying no. As Krista said, "I'm very, very happy with the way my life has gone, personally, professionally, and the interaction between those two. I'm glad I chose to be this version of me and my career."

Over the course of twelve years, Alan recognized and acted in ways that allowed him to craft a second career in medicine as part of the larger whole of his life and his values. He embraced agency in all its forms – saying no to his initial desire to do something big in medicine and to a career in academic medicine – and yes to the career path he enjoyed and that would sustain him. The last time we spoke, he said, "If you love the work – and if you see the work as important in and itself – it doesn't really matter how many hours you put into your work. You could work two or three hours a week and still be miserable." Alan's words resonate with the common adage, "Find the work you love, and you will never work again." But for Alan, finding the work he loved was not about which prestigious paths to pursue, but about which paths he needed to let go of.

CHAPTER 3

# Niki's Story About Balance

The road in the end taking the path the sun had taken,
into the western sea, and the moon rising behind you
as you stood where ground turned to ocean: no way
to your future now but the way your shadow could take,
walking before you across water, going where shadows go,
no way to make sense of a world that wouldn't let you pass
except to call an end to the way you had come,
to take out each frayed letter you brought
 and light their illumined corners; and to read
 them as they drifted through the western light;
 to empty your bags; to sort this and to leave that;
to promise what you needed to promise all along,
and to abandon the shoes that had brought you here
right at the water's edge, not because you had given up
 but because now, you would find a different way to tread,

and because, through it all, part of you could still walk on, no matter how, over the waves.

– David Whyte, "Finisterre"

David Whyte, "Finisterre," from *Pilgrim*. ©2014 David Whyte. Reprinted with permission from David Whyte and Many Rivers Company, LLC, Langley, WA. www.davidwhyte.com

## Introduction: "Where ground turned to ocean"

Niki lives life at lightning speed and makes every minute count. As a pediatrician, wife of a travel photographer, and mother of two young children, she has to. Not surprisingly, our calls often took place during a rare break in her day: her commute home from work. Those forty-five minutes were Niki's downtime. While the drive was necessary to get to and from work, it was also welcome. These were precious minutes that separated and buffered what happened at work from her life at home so that she could achieve a sense of balance between the two. "Driving home is my time to decompress from the day and let it all out," Niki told me in one of our last interviews. "The second I get home, I'm on again. I think of it like my day shift is my job, and my night shift is my family, especially when my husband is away." But balance for Niki did not mean that work and life outside of work were equal and opposing forces; indeed, often one would have to take precedence. Balance means that they were always in conversation with each other.[1]

Dialing back the years to when she was a fledgling medical student, Niki identified herself as a high achiever. She had graduated from an elite university and garnered the biomedical research experience that she needed for admission to an elite medical school. "For me, getting into this medical school is like a fulfillment of my goals because I have a checklist in my mind of where I want to be at each stage in my career, and in my life, and so far I've been able to check things off." Although Niki was able to keep up with the expectations that she had for herself for a while, she repeatedly discovered a need to revise her checklist and recalibrate her career goals – to find in David Whyte's words, "a different way to tread." How she responded to that need is the lesson of this chapter.

As the stories in this book reveal, the challenge of becoming a doctor is unrelenting. As a job, it's both exhilarating and stressful, filled with personal and professional highs and lows. The highs could be any number of things, from saving the life of a grandmother caught in the crossfire of a gang shooting to neatly stitching up the split chin of a boy who fell off a jungle gym. The lows can range from bone-rattling fatigue after a twenty-four-hour shift on the oncology floor to feeling as if one's efforts are futile when pronouncing the death of another teenager rushed into the emergency room after an overdose. But the stories aren't restricted to managing the challenge of becoming a doctor. The aspiring doctors in this book were also colleagues, life partners, siblings, parents, and much more. The real challenge was navigating all of life, including but not limited to medical training. Blake talked about the challenge like this:

> Part of what makes life and relationships hard with physicians is that sometimes you leave more of yourself at work than you take home with you. I feel like it really affects physician marriages, like they have higher divorce rates. It's really hard because you spend so much of your day giving to other people that you don't keep it for yourself. That is a very depressing thought, but it is a component of being a doctor ... it's definitely a balancing act between your career and your life.

Although it's no mystery that doctors experience a tremendous amount of stress over the course of their training, medical education has a fairly narrow conception of how to avoid becoming depleted and exhausted – what is frequently referred to as burnout. The research on burnout has evolved from seeing it as a problem that an individual doctor has to deal with to an occupational hazard that comes with the territory of being a doctor.[2] But largely missing in this shift of perspectives are the ways in which the doctors in this book dealt with stress as it manifested in their lives over time – not by merely trying to avoid burnout but by seeking a more elusive sense of balance in their lives as a whole.

Like all the other trainees featured in this book, Niki was eager to craft a successful career in medicine and become "the best" doctor she could be. Instead of thinking of "the best" along the usual lines of excellence in clinical practice or research productivity, or "the best" as academic pedigree like Eliza, she thought about being the best doctor in terms of how she could keep work in conversation with life outside of work. Different stressors would present themselves, and rather than simply avoiding burnout, Niki would regularly reset and realign her career goals so that she experienced an integrated sense of balance.

For Niki, there was not necessarily one thing to point to as explaining why this sense of balance mattered so much to her, but certainly an experience in her past loomed large in her thinking – her mother's nervous breakdown when she was in high school. She recalled:

> My mom was pulled in too many directions and didn't take time for herself. She had a high-power career, she had us kids, she had the church. It was too much for her. I saw her whole world fall apart and because her world fell apart, mine did too … From that, I learned that I can never *not* take self-care seriously. If I'm coming to breaking point and out of balance, I need to stop, reassess, and figure it out.

Witnessing the aftermath of her mom's mental health crisis made an indelible impression on Niki, but all of the aspiring doctors in this book were cognizant of the toll that medical training could take on their well-being. What is notable about Niki was her remarkable capacity to regularly stop in her tracks, consider her options, and then realign her goals. In doing so, she wasn't expecting to eradicate the highs and the lows of being a doctor, nor achieve some sort of idyllic personal existence. Rather, Niki's actions reveal her understanding that instead of merely seeking to avoid burnout, achieving a sense of balance would be a never-ending quest.

## "No way to make sense of a world": Rethinking burnout

To understand how doctors-in-training successfully navigate the demands of work and life outside of work, we have to understand what throws them off kilter. Many doctors today would blame burnout. Although physician burnout is not a new phenomenon, it has received widespread attention in recent years, particularly in the aftermath of COVID-19. At the same time, the understanding of the root cause of burnout has evolved. It is no longer viewed as an individual problem – an illness that can be cured – but more of an occupational hazard, something that can be managed by those on the job. For example, the National Academy of Medicine's Action Collaborative on Clinician Well-Being and Resilience describes the cause of burnout as "an imbalance" between "job demands and the available supportive resources in the organization."[3] The collaborative calls for redesigning clinical systems so that doctors have more support in managing the demands the profession puts on them. To monitor system changes, they rely heavily on tools to objectively measure burnout. In fact, burnout today has become synonymous with the Maslach Burnout Inventory and the three constructs it measures:

depersonalization, emotional exhaustion, and lack of personal accomplishment.[4]

However, some see medicine's response to burnout as too limited.[5] The work of social and organizational psychologist Ayala Pines frames the issue more holistically as affirming one's existence.[6] From her perspective, the burnout that doctors experience is neither an individual problem nor an occupational one but an imbalance between the meaning one derives from one's work and the demands of the workplace. In her view, doctors suffering from burnout are likely facing an existential crisis stemming from "our need to believe that our lives are meaningful and that the things we do – and consequently we ourselves – are useful and important."[7] As such, avoiding burnout at work is necessary but not sufficient for achieving balance. Balance points to not just a lack of meaning at work. It points to being out of touch with where and how one finds meaning in one's life as a whole.[8]

Conceptualizing burnout as an existential crisis helps to explain why burnout wasn't big enough to capture the stories medical trainees told over twelve years. Their stories in the context of the long arc of training reveal that balance is not the opposite of burnout but instead has a whole-life perspective, which includes work (and burnout at work), but is not only about what happens at work. Focusing only on burnout was insufficient because trainees were more than just doctors-in-training. But because medical educators have focused on burnout in time-limited, cross-sectional studies, often using objective measures, there is much we don't know about how trainees find careers that bring meaning to their lives and not just manage the demands of their work.

Achieving balance is no easy task, especially when viewed as an issue of finding meaning in one's life. And because people find meaning in life differently, they will define balance differently. Moreover, what is understood and experienced as balance at one stage of life may not be balanced in another context. And if achieving such balance is hard, measuring it is even harder; there is no Maslach Balance Inventory. In short, if what gives one's life meaning is highly idiomatic, subject to change through time, and dependent on context, then achieving balance isn't a one-and-done event, but rather a continuous process, an ongoing conversation filled with unpredictable twists and turns. As Niki's story illustrates, keeping life at work in conversation with life outside of work requires considerable finesse and continual refinement.

## "Take out each frayed letter": The challenge of information

When the doctors in this book were first-year medical students, it wasn't the demands of the workplace that created an imbalance – it was the demands of studying. They were expected to learn massive amounts of information, and they all echoed some version of the common analogy for the first year of medical school: "drinking from a firehose." Alan compared medical school to his other work experience:

> I knew that there was a huge amount of information, but to actually experience the mountain of knowledge that I am going to be picking away at for the next, well, for the rest of my life, even though I knew ahead of time, it's still a surprise to see just how much it is ... And that's pretty unique to medical school. There are few things in life that are this information-intense.

It might be surprising to hear that medical students felt overwhelmed by the amount of information they were expected to absorb. After all, successful medical school applicants were almost always successful high school and college students. This meant that they were already adept at absorbing high volumes of material. Nonetheless, some felt like they needed a break after college. For Niki, the mental break was necessary to recalibrate after a draining senior year of college: "I was fried. My plan was always to go to medical school, but I couldn't go straight through. I didn't think I'd make it. So I took the year to take a mental break, work on myself, and get healthy again physically and mentally."

Some of Niki's family members warned her that taking time off was risky – that if she took a break, she'd never go back to school. But she recognized that she needed to recharge if she was to have the stamina needed to get through medical school. The experience of her mother's nervous breakdown undoubtedly shaped her expectations in this regard and ultimately served her well. Refreshed after the year away from academics, Niki came to medical school "expecting like this magical place where we would learn exciting facts and that it would just be fun." But she soon acknowledged that though she was elated to be in medical school, it was still a lot of hard work, and there was no end to studying. The task at hand was learning to set boundaries. In that respect, Niki's experience with her mother meant she had a leg up on some of her peers. She'd go to bed when she was tired, not when she was done studying. It was an early lesson in balance that she would return to time and again.

## "Call an end to the way you had come": Discoveries during the clinical phase

Niki started medical school with a deep conviction about her choice of specialization: obstetrics and gynecology (OB-GYN). She had done research in OB-GYN to prepare for her intended career as an obstetrician and was certain that it was the right career for her. "I came in knowing exactly what I wanted to do," she said. "When I started medical school, I was like, I don't know about these people who are having questions about what they wanted to do; what's going on with them?" But Niki started having serious doubts when she was in her OB-GYN clerkship. As a specialty, OB-GYN is highly procedural, involving a lot of hands-on work, and she soon discovered that the procedures in OB-GYN weren't just delivering babies. There is a considerable amount of surgery involved, and not just cesarean sections. Much to her disappointment, she found that she really didn't like operating:

> I came to medical school to do OB-GYN, but now 100 per cent no way – *no way*. I'm not going to do that because I cannot do surgery. I shouldn't say I can't – I don't want to. I really, really, really don't want to, and that would be a very big, very important part of the job I thought I wanted. I still think it's a fascinating specialization, but it's not important enough to my life to have to do so much surgery.

A common adage among the doctors in this book when they were reflecting on early career plans was "I didn't know what I didn't know." In other words, there were things they could only learn about becoming a doctor from experience. Niki couldn't fully comprehend the amount of surgery involved in OB-GYN and just how much she disliked surgical procedures until she was "knee-deep" experiencing them. But her decision to opt out of OB-GYN had consequences that went far beyond respecting her distaste for surgery. It fundamentally thwarted her from achieving a career goal she'd set years before. She realized that the demands of working in OB-GYN were too great, and this led to a bout of burnout far worse when compared to her experience at the end of college:

> The college burnout was just "I need a break" before I keep going. Medical school burnout was so much worse because I was exhausted but didn't even *like* what I was doing. I had a quarter-life crisis. I was like, "What am I doing with my

life? I've been working my entire life toward a goal that now I don't even want."

At this critical juncture, without a career goal to guide her, Niki contemplated dropping out of medical school. She started out completely confident that she would pursue a career in OB-GYN, but now she was forced her to reconsider what meaning, if any, she would derive from her work as a doctor.

Instead of giving up on medicine altogether, Niki decided to recalibrate her goals. "I went in thinking I knew exactly what I wanted: you can't change me, you can't move me, you can't tell me anything else. But no – you can. You can change me. You can move me." She realized that she could alter her career direction to better align with what gave her meaning, and that realization was a huge relief:

> I realized I hadn't signed my name in blood anywhere saying that I had to do OB-GYN. The second I decided that I didn't really want to do it, I felt like a weight had been lifted off. I'm not responsible to anyone for doing OB-GYN. I can do whatever I want. I don't have to do this. No one's going to be upset with me if I decide I want to do something else.

Although unnerved by the realization that OB-GYN was not for her, Niki soon discovered a new passion. Her pediatrics rotation was the very last of her clerkship year and led her to a remarkable insight: "I was like, 'Oh, I didn't want to help people get pregnant. I wanted to take care of the babies after they come out. This makes so much sense to me now.'" Krista, another of the doctors in this book, had a similar experience of shifting from OB-GYN to pediatrics. But for Niki, her newfound interest in pediatrics was only part of it. More than OB-GYN (with its heavy dose of surgery), pediatrics had the potential to accommodate her need for balance, or as she said, "well-roundedness":

> These people [pediatricians] are very, very smart and on point. They get things done, but they're still very well-rounded. I think that comes from leadership in the Department of Pediatrics. They really care about you as a person and want faculty, staff, and residents to all be well-rounded people. They're leaders in their fields, yet they're so caring and have interests outside of the hospital.

The pediatricians Niki saw when she was a medical student were the whole package: they loved their work and worked hard at what they did, yet they could put it down at the end of the day and have a life outside of work. Moreover, they saw her as a person, not just a doctor-in-training. Niki was as committed to medicine as the other doctors in this book, but her prior life experiences oriented her toward keeping work in conversation with life outside of work. Avoiding burnout was not enough. She would have to create time and space for her interests outside of work to find the balance she needed.

In retrospect, Niki recognized her career change from OB-GYN to pediatrics as one of her "best life lessons" because it powerfully reinforced prioritizing balance over the achievement of "hard and fast" career goals. As a newly minted attending in pediatrics, she reflected on that lesson:

The letting go of OB-GYN and going toward pediatrics was difficult because that had been in my mind for so long. I had attached so much time and effort and energy and research to that. That was the toughest transition – being okay with doing something different than I had originally planned if it feels more balanced. Now I know I can make plans, but if plans change, that's okay.

## "Abandon the shoes that had brought you here": The trials of residency

For the aspiring doctors in this book, the stress of residency took the challenge of finding balance to a whole new level; work seemed to dominate all conversation. There was a dramatic change of focus from student-centric medical school to patient-centric residency. Residents were no longer just learners but employees with responsibilities for patient care. Niki described it as a complete switch in mindset:

> As a medical student, your mindset is very much, "I want to look good." That is all medical school is: looking good to get a good grade. But in residency, the focus is completely switched. It's about the patients, which is appropriate but hard to switch to that mindset.

Residents were not eased into this new phase of training, let alone eased into a new mindset. After a brief orientation, they jumped into the hospital trenches and worked long hours, often in high-volume and high-acuity patient care settings. Much like the information firehose at the start of medical school, Niki and her coresidents found themselves facing a patient care firehose, spending up to eighty hours a week at work. The results were predictably exhausting. Alan explained the fatigue caused by residency this way:

> You're always tired, always overworked. If you're at the end of a ten-day stretch working twelve hours a day and your patient codes and has to be rushed to the ICU, you just have to be on. You don't have any choice. You don't think about it. You just do it. You don't even have time to reflect on how tired you are.

Residency didn't just involve long hours. Those hours moved at a frantic pace, and so residents had to learn to work very efficiently. From the perspective of a first-year resident, everything seemed intense, even critical. For Niki, intensity meant "you can't turn it off," because as she explained, "When you are in the hospital, you really have to be observant of every little thing." She admitted that this attitude had started to seep into her personal life. "No matter what, you have to be efficient, you have to be organized, which has carried over to my personal life. My apartment has never been cleaner than when I was in residency!" In short, residency seemed antithetical to the kind of balance that Niki sought in her life.

In their attempts to keep work in conversation with life outside of work, residents found ways to maximize quality time with those they loved. But quality time could only go so far. Long hours at work meant they regularly missed out on birthdays, weddings, and other important life events. They neither had the time nor the energy for pastimes that they used to enjoy or things that brought restoration or beauty. There were Christmases and Thanksgivings where whole families were together, and they were the only one not there. Missing out on life events that cannot be repeated and not engaging in the things that used to bring them pleasure were real losses. "That wears on you after a while," Eliza shared. "You wonder if it will go on forever. That's when I ask myself, 'Is it worth it? As much as I love it, do I love it more than everything else in my life?'"

For the doctors in this book, the answer to that question was a version of "No, but ..." As their training dragged on, Niki and the others in this book struggled to make peace with being a resident. They regularly talked about buckling down and "powering through" the exhaustion they felt. They worked to get the work done, not because the work had meaning. Nor was it just physical exhaustion they felt. The mental and emotional fatigue was equally draining when encountering sudden illness, a tragic accident, and too often, untimely deaths. With every patient encounter, there was some story of pain and suffering. "Sometimes I would have nightmares about some of my patients, especially on the oncology rotation," Niki shared. "I talked to my colleagues, and they had the same experience. It was hard not to mentally take those kids home with you." At a particularly low point in his second year of residency, Blake divulged the toll residency was taking on him:

> I've been so burned out and busy with residency that I don't feel connected at all to that idealistic person that I was back in medical school. Honestly, it's painful to think about the goals I once had for my career and for my life. I feel like I can't hope to achieve them.

For Blake, residency came with dark and hopeless phases, but they were just that: phases. In fact, Blake chose his specialty because of the balance he thought it would offer in the long run. He just needed to get through residency:

> One of the things I saw in my specialty is that I could hope to have some work-life balance. But I think the nature of residency is not balanced, regardless of your specialty. I'm hoping it gets better. I'm hoping I see the light at the end of the tunnel, where I can create or at least find the right job that has the right balance for me.

To be clear, the long and arduous hours of residency were not problematic for everyone because balance meant different things to different people. Tim, a surgical resident, expected the hours to be long and wasn't deterred from surgery because of them. But even for him, the number of hours worked was only acceptable if he balanced those hours with what was needed to keep his "life and relationships outside of the hospital healthy":

> As a surgeon, my lifestyle is always going to be very demanding. And in some ways, I'm fine with that. I don't

mind working long hours, at least in the surgical world. I like what I am doing, and that's important to me. Getting lifestyle right, making sure I am present for home, my wife, my friends – that is still a challenge, and I haven't completely figured that out yet to be honest. But I'm fine working long hours in surgery. For me, it's about finding out how I can balance that in a way that keeps my life and my relationships outside the hospital healthy.

At various points in time, and depending on the training program, some residents were better resourced than others. But nothing brought home the significance of balance more than the knowledge that some residents became so burned out and unbalanced that they just wanted to end it all. Alan and Eliza mentioned the suicides of residents in programs in their region and expressed gratitude for the support their life partners gave them. Both suggested that doing a residency without a significant other was downright risky. Niki pointed out another source of support for residents: having a mentor who reminded them of the need to attend to their lives outside of work when they were in the thick of residency. Niki recalled the advice she received:

> I'd feel guilty if I didn't answer a clinic message within an hour, even if it was on a weekend. But my mentor would say, "You shouldn't feel guilty. To be the best doctor for your patients, you have to be a happy, healthy person. You can't neglect yourself or your family. You have to have friendships and a life outside of the hospital, or you can't really be a good doctor."

While it's one thing for a life partner or mentor to say, "Don't feel guilty about having a life outside the hospital," it's quite another for residents to truly embrace it – especially when medicine, on the whole, sees burnout as a problem that clinical systems can fix. Ultimately, residents had to internalize this lesson on their own timeline, and in their own way.

## "Find a different way to tread": A job versus a career

Niki graduated from pediatric residency and opted out of doing a fellowship in favor of taking a job as a primary care pediatrician. She was eager to jump right into the trenches and move forward with a new goal: tending not only to the physical but also the mental and social health of her patients, many of whom were from undocumented immigrant families. Niki felt a special connection to this group because she had aunts and uncles who were immigrants. She was well aware of their struggles to access healthcare, let alone to trust their healthcare providers:

> I feel like there is, in some cases, an unspoken understanding about things that you just can't get if you don't identify with immigrant families. There's this level of unspoken trust. I feel like families tend to open up to me, and I can be helpful in ways that other doctors cannot. It's not because I am better – but I have families who are undocumented immigrants, and they are scared to say *anything* to *anyone* about *anything*

at all. They don't want to draw attention to themselves. I talk to those families in their native language. If I'm able to communicate in their native language and share my personal story, it helps to make a safe space.

After a year working in pediatric primary care in an underserved neighborhood, Niki felt comfortable with her clinical skills. She saw lots of patients who needed the services she could provide. But she also stayed late into the evening to make phone calls, coordinate care, and complete the paperwork necessary to advocate for her patients' behalf. Over time, the workload of primary care took a toll on the balance she sought. Despite her best intentions to care for the physical, mental, and social needs of her patients, she realized that there were some things she couldn't do and some kids she couldn't help. "What I've learned is kind of depressing: you can't save everyone," Niki admitted. Recalling the essential lesson that she had learned from what happened to her mother, she knew it was time to recalibrate: "I really need work-life balance. I can't just work around the clock. So now I leave work at work, and when I'm home, I'm home. I'm doing the best I can and trying to be okay with that."

Niki stayed in her job in primary care pediatrics for another year. Although she had high regard for her team and a commitment to working with immigrant families, the combination of workload and feelings of guilt around recognizing "you can't save everyone" were untenable. To top things off, she and her husband were eager to start a family. She came to the realization that at this point in her life, raising a family was her priority – not work. "My husband and I are planning our lives around our family. My job will be something secondary that I do. Don't get me wrong; being a doctor will fulfill me and give me joy. But my family life will take precedence." And so Niki started looking for another job that would offer the sense of balance that she sought for her life – at this juncture.

In considering her options, Niki returned to an interest she had explored as a resident: school-based health.[9] Although her pediatric residency program (like most others) was inpatient-heavy and acute-care oriented, it did expose residents to pediatricians in outpatient settings. On one such occasion, Niki shadowed a pediatrician working in public schools and found it so interesting that she partnered with her residency program director to create an elective rotation in school health for other residents. She even interviewed for a position in school health when she graduated from residency but decided to try primary care first. In her mind, pediatric primary care would provide a broad foundation, and she could always step into school health from there. Now with primary care behind her, she was ready to move on and do something different than originally planned – all in the ongoing struggle to keep work in conversation with life outside of work.

Niki found a position in school health, and after just a few short months on the job, she knew she was in the right place. Her work enabled her to be an advocate for children's physical, mental, and social health in ways that she could not in primary care. For example, on occasion Niki had to tell teenage girls that they were pregnant. This task was not unique to school health, but in this context, she could help girls reach the best decision for them, free of coercion from the fathers, their parents, or their friends. Niki compared her care for pregnant teenagers in a school setting to what she could and couldn't do in primary care:

> It's a completely different kind of medicine. You are changing these kids' lives, being able to be there in the school and give them free confidential services. To be honest, I'm like a mother figure for a lot of these girls because they don't have anyone else to talk to. In school, I can say, "You know what? Why don't you come back tomorrow, and we'll talk about it some more." In primary care, you have to bring them physically into the clinic during your office hours, and their parents are going to know. So now, not feeling any pressure for time, having these intense conversations in private, and being able to develop relationships – you can really affect these girls' lives.

Niki's life lesson from medical school about being okay if plans change again paid dividends when COVID-19 turned everything upside down. Schools were closed due to public health mandates, and Niki found herself pulled into a role supervising the occupational health hotline for a regional hospital. Initially frustrated by the lack of a pediatric job, she had a patient encounter that helped her reframe her thinking. At the beginning of the pandemic when COVID-related hospitalizations and death rates were rising exponentially, a woman called the hotline, saying she couldn't come to work because her oxygen was very low, but she couldn't go to the hospital either because she was home alone with her infant daughter. Niki, herself six months pregnant, worked diligently to comfort this woman and provide the resources she needed. This harrowing experience brought her back to finding meaning in work – to be versatile and helpful to all people – even if it wasn't exactly the job she anticipated.

Nonetheless, when it comes to balance, finding meaning in work is not enough. One needs to find meaning in life outside of work. Niki eventually returned to school health, not only because it was meaningful work, but also because it was a flexible workplace with reasonable demands on her time. She was clear that she didn't want an all-encompassing career in medicine – at this point in her life. From her vantage point, that was not being the best doctor she could be. What Niki wanted was a job that allowed her "to go home every day and say, 'I made a difference' and be happy and not be totally overwhelmed." Working in school health meant dealing with relatively healthy kids and having predictable daytime hours, Monday through Friday, with plenty of scheduled vacation and summers off.

## "To your future now": The role of family

Niki's drive for balance in the present was not only shaped by her past, but it also shaped her future. She was planning her life around her family, not around her career. She was very happy in school health and had no plans not to work. But when she was home, she wanted to be fully present. "I'm not even thinking about progressing in terms of my career. I'm just focusing on home and family." Fast forward two years to find Niki with a toddler in tow and another baby on the way. She looked back on her decision to move into school health as one of the best decisions she ever made. Her work had meaning. And she was able to prioritize her family.

> My career is totally on the back burner right now, which I never thought would happen to me when I was in medical school. My family is just much more important to me right now. Once the kids are in school and I get bored, maybe that will change. But right now, my job is not as important to me as what is happening at home.

But that didn't mean that keeping work in conversation with life outside of work was easy. The arrival of a second child meant more responsibilities at home. She heightened her resolve and "divorced" her work from her home life.

> I work really hard not to bring the cases home with me because literally the second I walk in the door I have kids jumping on me. There's no break; there's no off button. I have to be present for my children the minute I walk in the door. It's impossible not to have it affect you at all, but I've worked really hard to divorce myself for the sake of my patients and for the sake of my children.

Niki wasn't the only doctor in this book whose outlook on balancing work with life outside of work changed when children came on the scene. Tim was caught off guard by how much a newborn could challenge the prioritization of work: "I had this stark moment of realization once I had my daughter. I totally regretted not being sensitive to my peers who had kids when I was in residency and was responsible for scheduling. I had some control over their lives but didn't know how excruciating it is to balance surgical training with having a family."

## Conclusion: "Still walk on"

The saying "coming full circle" nicely sums up Niki's story. When she started medical school, she was convinced she'd be in OB-GYN, only to pivot to pediatric primary care before finally winding up in school-based health. In her career's latest twist, Niki ironically became an adolescent reproductive health specialist, not unlike an OB-GYN for teenagers. Niki smiled as she explained this twist:

> I've become the go-to reproductive specialist for the school district. I don't know how I ended up here from wanting to be in OB-GYN to now being an adolescent reproductive specialist, but that's what happened! What I do is really important, and I feel really good about it. I just needed to tweak my goals to end up in the right place for me.

Niki's career goals had changed in response to different stressors that threatened to throw her off-kilter or even out of medicine. She and the other doctors in this book consistently sought ways to avoid burnout; that was necessary but not sufficient. Over the long arc of training, they learned to pay close attention to how they were – or were not – living their whole lives, examining their careers, family lives, health, and personal interests with more nuance than can be found in a vague concept of work-life balance. With regular reflection and refinement, they, like Niki, would end up in the right place for them.

CHAPTER 4

# Krista's Story About Emotion

And a woman spoke, saying, Tell us of Pain.
And he said:
Your pain is the breaking of the shell that encloses your understanding.
Even as the stone of the fruit must break, that its heart may stand in the sun, so must you know pain.
And could you keep your heart in wonder at the daily miracles of your life, your pain would not seem less wondrous than your joy;
And you would accept the seasons of your heart, even as you have always accepted the seasons that pass over your fields.
And you would watch with serenity through the winters of your grief.
Much of your pain is self-chosen.
It is the bitter potion by which the physician within you heals your sick self.

Therefore trust the physician, and drink his remedy in silence and tranquility:
For his hand, though heavy and hard, is guided by the tender hand of the Unseen,
And the cup he brings, though it burn your lips, has been fashioned of the clay which the Potter has moistened with His own sacred tears.
– Kahlil Gibran, "On Pain," *The Prophet*

## Introduction: "Tell us of Pain"

Most of my interviews with Krista took place outside in late spring or early summer, with her sitting on a porch or in a park, soaking up the sun. That setting is wholly appropriate, as it matches the warmth of Krista's personality. She was fervent in her quest to become a doctor and enamored by the depth of human care and connection that a career in medicine would afford. And even though things got hard as her training progressed, Krista kept her grip on that deep emotional anchor that grounded her truest self: "Anytime I get a high five from my patient, that's a win. Or I'll just get spontaneous hugs from my clinic patients and then it's like, that is the best thing ever."

Much like the warmth of spring morphs into the heat of summer, which then evolves into the crispness of fall and the frigidness of winter, so too do the emotions of medical trainees evolve. But the change of seasons is too slow an analogy. Krista came up with a better one, explaining that doctors are asked to wear many emotional hats. They are expected to be healers who feel compassion but not aggravation, clinicians who feel sadness but not anguish, and health advocates who feel passionate but not hopeless. They are expected to feel (or not to feel) these emotions like they were wearing a top hat in one patient encounter and then swapping it out for a baseball cap in the next. Once, when Krista was an intern, she wondered how she could have a "bad day" when some of her patients needed her to be optimistic. It seemed there was little space for her emotions:

> If I'm in a bad mood or if something bad is happening outside of work, you learn to compartmentalize. Or to least you learn to kind of say, "Yes, okay things are not so great, but I have a patient in front of me who deserves my attention and my emotional energy." And you learn to at least try to have that give way to the demands of what you are doing.

Krista was not alone. All of the aspiring doctors in this book grappled with managing their emotions. They would all know pain. For example, Alan talked about reaching the limits of his emotional reserve after seeing things like men his age die while doctors were trying to resuscitate them.

> These are basically unavoidable things, and I've learned that I can think about them in technical terms. Before I started residency, I had the mindset that people who weren't deeply emotionally affected by these things were probably suppressing it unhealthily. Or that it was a negative trait. But I've come to a point where I can, or at least I have – I don't know if it's good or bad – been able to think about them in non-emotional terms.

As Krista later articulated, there were two options: doctors-in-training could compartmentalize emotions and put them at a distance, or they could acknowledge emotions and try to manage how they felt in the moment. Neither option was right or wrong, and neither was uniformly recommended by the doctors in this book. They had to figure out how to manage intense emotions pretty much on their own, even though there was starting to be an uptick in physician wellness resources by the time the doctors in this book were in training.

Trainees' tendency to go it alone was notable in terms of managing emotions, but so too was the striking disconnect between the wide range of emotions that they felt and the narrow coverage of emotions in medical education. For example, literature describes how medical students are taught "to do" empathy in patient encounters – that is, how to communicate empathically, how to listen empathically, and even how to act empathically.[1] To be clear, Krista spoke movingly of empathizing with her patients, trying to understand their feelings, thoughts, and experiences. But she experienced a range of emotions beyond just empathy that both surprised her and caused her to reflect on the importance of emotions in becoming a doctor. This chapter goes further than the well-trodden ground on empathy to look at a range of intense emotions that routinely surface over the long arc of medical training.

Krista's story is particularly illustrative of the role that emotions play in the process of becoming a doctor. She was drawn to role-playing games such as Dungeons and Dragons as a young adult because they afford players emotional experiences they might not otherwise have, such as exulting in casting down a tyrannical villain or reveling in the naughtiness of robbing the king blind. While role-playing games can be emotionally intense, players have a safe space to explore those emotions. These games were intriguing while Krista was in medical school, as they supplemented what she was learning about empathy in the classroom. But residency changed things. Emotional intensity was no longer a game – it was real life: "The stresses of where I'm at in residency have conspired to really make me look with new eyes and from a new point of view of how I function." Intense emotions in the daily course of work meant that Krista no longer had the bandwidth for role-playing games. Like the other doctors in this book, she had to figure out how to manage emotions in her day-to-day life at work – and life outside of work.

## "Breaking of the shell that encloses your understanding": The work of emotions

There is an extensive literature on emotions, but for the purposes of this chapter I draw from Arlie Hochschild's research on emotion work, which she defines as a socially situated act of shaping an emotion in oneself.[2] Emotion work is distinguished from emotional labor, which is a public act of evoking, shaping, or suppressing emotion as part of one's job.[3] While emotional labor could be considered part of the job of being a doctor, and thus a worthwhile part of their formal training, in tracing Krista's story I've focused on how doctors informally learn to manage their own emotions over the course of their training. Managing their emotions wasn't a performance, and it wasn't trying to quelch any emotion that suddenly appeared. It was learning to acknowledge one's emotions and notice when emotions seemed appropriate in any given social situation.

Some view emotions as a reflex and part of our physical makeup. As Hochschild points out, because emotions seem "unbidden and uncontrollable," they are often characterized as being almost instinctual.[4] Others view emotions as a social performance that can be developed through practice.[5] But a closer examination of emotions reveals them to be much more malleable than the picture typically painted of them as sprouting up or directed by social rules. Emotion work is what people are doing when they are trying *not* to feel or constraining themselves when they feel *too much*. When Krista made comments like she couldn't allow herself to feel both joy and grief at the same time, she was doing emotion work. When she talked about how to provide emotional self-care and compassionate patient care at the same time, she was doing emotion work. In essence, doing emotion work was part and parcel of doing the work of a doctor.

Another way to think about what's happening in these situations is the notion of emotional agility. People rarely give their emotions free rein, particularly in professional settings. Instead, they seek to manage emotions by inducing a range of feelings that are viewed as appropriate or by inhibiting other feelings that are viewed as inappropriate. A feeling's appropriateness is determined by *feeling rules* derived from socio-cultural forces that tell us how we should feel in any given situation.[6] Feeling rules trigger the management of emotions, not the management of social performances. This internal work of managing emotions is most apparent when our feelings do not fit the situation – that is, when feeling rules do not legitimate the feelings we actually have. For example, an event, such as a patient's death, often carries with it a proper definition of itself ("this is a time of facing loss"). But what happens when inner emotions clash with feeling rules? What happens when doctors not only feel sadness for the loss but also relief that there is one less patient they must manage?

In medical education, we know little about the broader phenomenon of emotion work and how it changes over the course of training. Learning about this requires a longitudinal approach to capture the complex emotional ups and downs of doctors-in-training. Instead, medical education has focused on empathy and often reduced it to a measurable variable with tools like the Jefferson Scale of Physician Empathy.[7] Research using static measures like surveys suggests that, despite all the effort made to teach students empathy, it declines over the course of medical training.[8] And so medical students assume their empathy will decline, and are coached on how to act empathic even if they don't necessarily feel it. But what if they instead are taught to expect an ebb and flow of empathy, and not a steady decline? And what about the host of other emotions (and often conflicting emotions) they experience over the long arc of training? The bigger issue at hand seems to be how to help aspiring doctors figure out how to manage a whole range of emotions, including but not limited to empathy.

## "So must you know pain": Emotions and the journey to medicine

Like the other doctors in this book, Krista was at the top of her class in high school and college. She started as a biology major, but when she got a B+ in organic chemistry after acing every other science course since high school, she took a sharp turn: "It was traumatizing ... I was like, Oh my God, what's happening? I can't do this." So, she didn't. Krista switched her college major to history. Toward the end of her junior year in college, she had another disorienting experience when she realized that she didn't want to do any of the jobs that were traditionally open to history majors. In response, Krista "went on this wild career exploration." She ultimately returned to science and settled on medicine, inspired by her mother's advice to capitalize on her interest in women's issues and pursue women's health.

While Krista was taking the prerequisite college courses for medical school, she heard about a new program that offered an alternative path for clerkships. Instead of the traditional block rotations over the course of year, the new program had a longitudinal integrated clerkship where medical students follow their own diverse panel of patients. Students moved with patients through different clinical specialties over twelve months. They got to know patients and their families as people and saw their medical care as process, not as points in time. That's what made the new program perfect for Krista:

> I think the biggest draw for me personally was the focus on relationships, that longitudinal patient care experience. One of the reasons I decided to go into medicine was because I wanted that kind of direct human involvement.

What mattered to Krista was getting to know patients as people and not just individuals with medical conditions. More than snapshot encounters, the longitudinal relationships would afford Krista the opportunity to deepen human connections with patients – and experience the types of intense emotions that these connections tend to elicit.

## "Keep your heart in wonder": Empathy and medical school

Krista anticipated that the basic sciences like histology, pathology, and gross anatomy would be the most difficult part of medical school because she wasn't a science major all the way through college: "I was nervous that all of these science people were going to blow right past me and I was going to be lost." While studying basic sciences did consume most of Krista's time in the first year of medical school, other classes introduced the art of clinical medicine. As part of a foundational doctoring course in the pre-clerkship phase, students worked in small groups to learn how to interview and do physical exams on hospitalized patients. They then met with an attending physician who served as their clinical preceptor and discussed the patient they had just seen. But medical students learned much more than history-taking and physical exam skills in their doctoring course. They learned about the personal, psychosocial, and societal aspects of illness that add to the complexity of clinical medicine. And they learned communication strategies necessary to build relationships with patients and families, taking into account the non-clinical aspects of illness. Part of relationship building entailed learning how to convey empathy – that is, listening to and understanding the patient's perspective, communicating that understanding, and acting in a way that was helpful by expressing care, respect, and support.[9]

It might sound surprising, but there is a robust debate about whether empathy can be effectively taught. Even Krista had her doubts, noting that empathy was "not a science" – rather, it was something that students were expected to come into medicine with. In her words, "It's still considered less of a skill and more of something that either just happens or you should have." Nonetheless, students essentially were taught how to be empathic in their interactions with patients, or how to "do empathy," often by practicing with standardized patients – actors who were trained to portray patient scenarios and to give feedback that students could use to improve empathic communication and actions. Despite regularly engaging in role-playing games to satisfy her yearning to explore emotions, Krista was surprised by how emotionally fraught it was to practice with a standardized patient:

> I had to tell the standardized patient that she had cancer; she started crying, and I almost started crying. It was actually

really intense. Normally in the class interviews with standardized patients, you're very conscious of the people who are watching you – or at least I am. But when I was talking to this standardized patient, it was complete tunnel vision. All I saw was her, and it was so much harder than I thought.

But much like how standardized patients are not real patients, medical students are not real doctors. Many of Krista's classmates felt that acting the part of a doctor translated to merely acting empathic. Niki, for one, doubted the genuineness of that empathy: "I feel strongly that they are teaching us to put on a good show. I had a preceptor say to me, 'You do a really good job of pretending and, like, showing empathy. By the time you're where I am, you'll be so good at putting on an act that it will just feel natural.'"

Perhaps because students like Niki questioned the authenticity of acting empathic (particularly when being assessed by medical school faculty), they worried about not being able to sustain empathy in medical training. For instance, Eliza remarked, "If I can remember that I need to see people as people and remember that that's important to me, I'll be okay. Otherwise, I've really failed myself as a physician." Their worries were not unfounded. A trope in medical education is that empathy declines over the course of their arduous training. All of the aspiring doctors in this book were cognizant of this. As a first-year medical student, Krista voiced optimism that she could resist becoming cynical:

In a general, idealistic medical student kind of way, I would hope that we will all be able to maintain our perhaps more humanistic side – I mean all the stuff we are learning now about empathy in the doctoring course. The stereotype is that you have all these idealistic medical students, and then they go out and become jaded practitioners.

Over a decade later when she was looking in the rearview mirror, Krista pushed back on the trope:

The stereotype is that when you are a med student you are this bleeding heart and that you care so much. Then it gets beaten out of you by medical training. But my friends from medical school and I were talking this weekend, and that has not been what's happened to us. We have become more vulnerable to feeling empathy or feeling like we are just trying to help. We talk a lot about, like, how you feel that and what you do for yourself in order to make it feasible and sustainable?

From this more experienced vantage point, Krista mused on the meaning of empathy. She didn't believe she could really know what someone else was feeling, thinking, or experiencing. So the best she could do is to be "good": "When I think about what I'm doing for patients and families, it's not that I am providing empathy. I'm hoping that in the context of what could be the worst thing that ever happened to them, I'm just being good to them."

None of the doctors in this book mentioned explicit teaching on how to manage their emotions beyond evoking empathy. This is not to say that they were never taught how to navigate emotionally stressful situations. But when they talked about these situations, they never referred back to explicit teaching. Instead, they grappled with their feelings through personal reflection and informal conversations with peers and family, often expressing guilt about their emotional reactions. For instance, Krista herself admitted, "It feels uncharitable to get so frustrated when you see patients with chronic diseases like diabetes who come into the hospital at least once a month because maybe they can't take care of themselves, or maybe they are unwilling to. I know it's not their fault, but it still gets at me."

## "Accept the seasons of your heart": The range of emotions during clerkship

In line with her penchant for role-playing games, Krista purposefully sought out intense emotional experiences in ways that others did not. In her words, these intense emotions were "what makes me tick." Not surprisingly, she wholeheartedly engaged in some of life's most momentous occasions in her clerkship year. Her stories about longitudinal relationships with patients, afforded by her participation in a longitudinal integrated clerkship, reverberated with emotion. One was about a patient she cared for in the Emergency Department: a woman who was thirty-five weeks pregnant and in pain. The nurses feared that the patient (whom I'll call Kelly) would deliver, so they wanted to transfer her to the maternity ward. However, Krista was sure Kelly was in extreme pain, not labor. She sat with Kelly for over an hour, talking her through the pain and waiting for the pain medication to take effect. In the process, Krista learned about Kelly's need for social support and later connected Kelly to the appropriate resources. Given the longitudinal structure of her clerkship, Krista was able to check in with Kelly at her subsequent prenatal visits – "not only from a medical standpoint but from a social standpoint." She gave Kelly her pager number so that she could contact her when she went into labor. Krista recalled responding quickly to Kelly's page:

> I got to the hospital within ten minutes. It was like twelve hours of labor, and I was there most of the time. I ended up being the one to catch her baby. I sewed up her lacerations. I delivered the placenta. And then afterward her partner was taking pictures, and I asked, "Do you want me to take a picture of you two with the baby?" Kelly was like, "I want one with you and the baby. You've done so much for us that we're changing her middle name to Krista, to be named after you."

Undoubtedly, there is not one right way to manage one's emotions, and individuals manage emotions differently. Blake was in the same longitudinal integrated clerkship as Krista but had a different experience. He described himself as empathic, but rather than medical school being a hotbed for emotions, for him it was emotionally barren:

> I think I have empathy at a baseline, but often I've felt like it was a part that I was ignoring. In medical school, the focus is always on answering the question right or putting in the right orders or whatever. It's just the day-to-day stuff that makes it easy to ignore my empathetic side.

For Krista, the last few months of medical school were fraught with a different type of intense emotional experience – one focused not on her patients, but on her career. Despite being told she had a very strong residency application, Krista didn't match into the residency program that she wanted. That rarely happens for graduates of elite medical schools like the one Krista attended. The effect can be devastating emotionally, and there are doctors who thirty years after the fact can still vividly describe the shock of the match not working out as they had hoped. For Krista, it was "the biggest upset of my professional career." As she went on to explain,

> Dealing with that was very difficult. I was fortunate that up until that point I really hadn't experienced any significant academic or professional failure. Now I acknowledge that the result was probably the best possible outcome. But at the time and for the first year afterward, I really struggled with feeling like I had a place and knowing where my place was. It was a big hit to my ego, to be very frank. It definitely complicated my transition to residency.

Krista's experience with the match reminds us that emotion work is not limited to patient encounters in the hospital. Krista struggled to know how to manage emotions evoked by professional failure (or at least what she perceived as such at the time). It wasn't just "a radical reconceptualization of who I was" – it was changing how she felt, much like trying to smile to change one's emotions.

## "Watch with serenity through the winters of your grief": The difficult emotions in residency

Residency took emotion work to a whole different level. As medical students, the aspiring doctors in this book encountered rules around "doing empathy." In residency, they encountered rules around not catering to their own emotions. Recall that when Krista was in medical school, she had the bandwidth to manage emotions evoked through role-playing games. But emotion work was different in residency because it felt closer, more real. She was no longer approximating the role of a doctor. She had the initials "MD" behind her name:

> I don't feel like the demands of residency are a different beast than the demands of medical school. They're just more intense because there's one less layer of an alibi. You can't say, oh, I'm just a student. This is my job now. So there's, like, one less layer of separation between you and the patient.

Residents were still medical trainees – still learners – but not only students. As we learned in prior chapters, residency was both a workplace and a "clinical classroom." Residents were trainees but also paid employees and a critical part of the workforce of hospitals. As such, residents routinely talked about feeling more responsible for patients when they transitioned from medical school to residency. But responsibility wasn't just understood as being accountable for patient care. Responsibility carried a significant emotional element that needed to be managed with respect to patients' well-being. For instance, Blake recalled that as a medical student, he followed patients and was involved in their care. But he didn't feel liable for every aspect of their care: "As a medical student, you're there and you're a part of it, but ultimately, it's someone else's responsibility to make sure things get done." He contrasted what it was like following patients in medical school with the acute responsibility he felt in residency:

> Being an intern is a big transition and part of it is seeing myself as a doctor and taking ownership of my patients. I didn't feel as much of the ownership of it as a medical student. But now it is all on me.

To be clear, residents were under the supervision of attending physicians who were ultimately responsible for patient care. But that did not diminish the sense of responsibility that residents felt for their patients. They wanted the best for their patients, but there were limits on how much they could pour into their work before they broke down. Eliza described it this way: "You could let things go, but then there is the shame factor. How much can I do before I feel ashamed that I didn't do it? You find out how much you can give before you break."

Each doctor in this book had their own limits on how much emotional energy they could extend. What is more, they went into different specialties and trained at different residency programs with different socio-cultural forces that constructed different feeling rules. Krista understood that her emotional side was part of who she was; it shaped her sense of self as a doctor. Her emotions were something to celebrate, but they were also something to manage:

> There is definitely a wide range of emotions, even among my coresidents ... some people are calmer than others, and some people just go with the flow more easily than others. I tend to be more on the emotional side. I've become a lot better over the years – not so much in terms of not being emotional but in controlling how my emotions present to the world.

For the sake of her patients and junior colleagues, Krista believed she had to present herself as strong. In her words, "I can't indulge in all of my emotions, at least not publicly." It wasn't that she couldn't feel some emotions – she just couldn't freely act on them in social spaces: "I definitely don't want to lose that emotional side of myself. But I know that in order to make those around me feel comfortable, I'm going to have to present myself as a source of strength to them." Still, some scenarios challenged this feeling rule about not catering to one's emotions in public. Krista recalled a specific encounter in her second year of residency:

> On another occasion, I was in the Emergency Department, and we had this baby come in who ended up coding, and it was a really, really bad end-of-life experience, like an hour and a half of active code that was unsuccessful. I remember when I finally went out of that patient's room where the family was in there crying, and I went to check on one of my other patients who I had not seen for an hour and a half, and

> I was still crying – this was a patient I had known intermittently for all of his life – and the mother ended up really very genuinely comforting me, which was an odd experience … When I was talking about it afterward, I realized that it is normal and inherently human to comfort somebody who is in distress or grieving. But then you realize how odd it is to think that it is odd to be comforted. Or how odd it is to be the one who is comforted.

Krista's recollection of the time a patient's mother ended up comforting her is anything but odd: seeing another person grieve is a social situation that legitimizes extending comfort because care and connection are central to our human nature. Yet when she was in residency, Krista had to go through mental gymnastics to see it as such.

Toward the end of her residency, Krista spoke poignantly of managing her emotions as wearing different emotional hats. She had learned to be emotionally agile. In one room, she was genuinely happy for a young patient with a complicated medical history who was recovering from surgery much better than anyone had expected. In the next room, she was genuinely grieving with a family whose daughter had just died in a car accident.

> Having to flip back and forth so rapidly – you learn that, even if you can't process emotions in the moment … Every time you walk into a patient's room you have to be able to read what the patient or family wants from you and to some extent or another when it's appropriate, provide that for them, whether it is mutual concern or excitement or grief.

Krista went on to explain that it wasn't suppressing emotion so much as not letting the emotions evoked by one patient spill over to another: "You learn to have whatever emotions you are feeling underneath it all, but as much as possible, you don't let those emotions affect what you are doing when you go in to see that next patient." By wearing different emotional hats, Krista had not lost her capacity to feel emotions. She wasn't compartmentalizing or detaching so as not to feel emotion. She was just better at managing her emotions so that she had enough emotional capacity to be the kind of doctor she wanted to be for all of her patients, no matter what the situation.

In the context of medical training, emotion work wasn't just dealing with the diversity of emotions; it was also the pace. Reminiscent of Niki and the challenge to find a glimmer of balance in residency, the sheer volume of patients that residents cared for meant that they couldn't stay in any one emotion for too long, and the accumulation of patient experiences made it hard for any one emotional experience to stand out. However, for Krista, this didn't diminish the emotional intensity of what she felt: "I don't feel like those individual patient experiences have become any less meaningful. It's just that there are more of them. You lose some of that acute stress reaction, but it does not lose its emotional valence."

To be sure, not every aspiring doctor in this book managed emotions like Krista. For example, in contrast to Krista's tendency to shape emotions, Tim, a surgical resident, spoke of emotion work more passively. He specifically referred to emotional distancing as something that happened to him almost as if he had been vaccinated. It was like dealing with emotions early in his internship was a pathogen that stimulated emotional remove:

> I've spontaneously found that emotional distance isn't a coping mechanism or in any way unhealthy psychologically. That surprised me a little bit. I guess I learned to be emotionally distant through inoculation, in a way. The first couple of times something bad would happen, I'd think, "This should be making a big emotional mark on me." But after it happened a couple more times and the year progressed, it became less important that bad outcomes occurred because you learn this is part of the pace of surgery.

This is not to say that Tim always compartmentalized and never wore different emotional hats or that Krista never felt emotionally distant. Later in training, Krista shared how easy it was to "fall into moments of compassion fatigue" by referring to patients by their diagnosis and not their name or casting difficult parents into the "bad guy" role. Even Tim found himself bound up in intense emotions. He shared this story about a young patient with a fairly benign cancer, but whose preexisting medical issues became life-limiting issues post-operatively:

> She ultimately succumbed in a few weeks. I think what made it most gut-wrenching was that, toward the end, there was this kind of palpable feeling that we weren't going to get her through this. But she was very young, and so we were as aggressive as possible. But there was a kind of sense of futility ... it was a very emotionally challenging situation ... On most rotations, we only see portions of patients' trajectories.

Even when they're having a kind of downward trajectory, we might come in midway through, or leave before it reaches its culmination. But this time, I started the rotation, you know, and within a couple of days, we did her initial surgery and I saw her entire course and managed it throughout ... so you know, it was very challenging, but also kind of instructive in a way, in terms of the emotional turmoil that surgical complications can have on you.

Tim's story is compelling because, much like Krista's experience in a longitudinal integrated clerkship, he acknowledged the lasting impact of longitudinal relationships with patients – of being with a patient from the initial surgery through the end. What started out as feelings of hope – young patient, benign cancer – turned over the course of a few weeks into feelings of futility. Yet these types of longitudinal relationships were not the norm in medical training. Most patient relationships were fleeting encounters that did little to expose trainees to the emotional turmoil Tim mentioned, much less offer opportunities to learn how to navigate intense emotions.

## "The physician within you heals your sick self": Emotional discoveries during fellowship

Krista was unique among the doctors in this book in that she served as a staff physician and frontline provider for a few years between residency and fellowship. In her case, she worked with a team of neonatology attendings, neonatology fellows, and advanced practice nurses in a neonatal intensive care unit. This type of job provided a viable alternative to going directly into a neonatology fellowship after residency, allowing her to test out her interest in this subspeciality of pediatrics and take a break from formal training. During her two years as a frontline provider, she and her husband (also a physician) often reflected back on their experience as medical trainees and pondered "what medical education has done to us." This was a type of retrospective emotion work, as their discussions delved into the emotional aspects of what they had experienced. Krista offered this summary of their conversations and how they felt:

> It's almost a trauma that's inherent to medical education ... It's like you are up against a behemoth. It's kind of hard to feel sometimes like you have any power to change it.

Taking a frontline provider position also afforded Krista some time to consider what type of career she wanted in neonatology. Unlike some specialties with few employment options outside of academic medical centers, neonatologists can work in smaller community hospitals or private practice for large healthcare companies. Krista reflected on her interests in college and medical school and decided to recommit to an academic career:

> I'm in a very different place compared to a year ago. I was thinking that I would end up being the clinically working

breadwinner to support my husband's academic career. But I've had time to think about who I am and what I want. I realized that an academic career is also what I want for me. It's not like only one of us gets to do that. We can both do that, or at least attempt it.

Armed with two years of experience from her staff position, Krista had solid clinical skills and defined research interests when she applied for a fellowship at several research-intensive, academic institutions. In contrast to what happened for her residency match, she got the competitive fellowship she wanted. The real challenge in fellowship was that, like Eliza, she chose to do a master's degree in an adjacent field to biomedical science – bioethics. But studying and responding to moral and ethical questions in medicine spoke to Krista's proclivity for intense emotions. Despite one of her fellowship directors expressing concern about getting a degree that few in biomedical science would recognize, Krista persisted:

> I'm just really actually proud of myself for my determination to make this work because it wasn't what other fellows did. I've spent a lot of time and emotional energy trying to figure out ways to make this happen. I feel like, if nothing else, I've proven that I really want this degree.

Krista pursued the master's degree she wanted, but her neonatal fellowship itself wasn't entirely smooth sailing. The COVID-19 pandemic happened, and with it all kinds of precautions like the donning and doffing of personal protective equipment as a routine part of patient care and moving didactics to an online learning platform. To top it off, Krista was pregnant during her second year of fellowship, which presented its own unique emotional challenges. She encountered "odd experiences" like doing chest compressions on a critically ill newborn while having prodromal labor or being asked to talk to the parents of a very premature baby who had opted for comfort care versus aggressive resuscitation at a time during her own pregnancy when, had Krista gone into labor, she would have given birth to a child at the same gestational age.

At the end of her fellowship and on the precipice of being an attending neonatologist, Krista revisited her emotional hats metaphor, offering another dimension to her understanding of how she came at emotion work:

> What wearing different emotional hats misses is that all of these emotions are real. When I go in and share grief or celebrate with a family, all of those are real things that I am feeling. What I have made a point of doing and modeling is taking a moment after bad things happen, not just immediately moving on to the next thing. I take a moment and give myself some emotional space, not trying to pretend that things are all good or pretend to be happy. It's feeling the things you are feeling and moving forward, not suppressing things but saying, "Yes, this is the moment I am in right now. I'm honoring this feeling now and then moving on when I will feel something else."

For Krista, emotion work was a lot more than simply "doing empathy." And she found ways to feel a range of emotions without giving up parts of herself that made her the doctor she was.

## Conclusion: "His own sacred tears"

Like other aspiring doctors in this book, Krista had grown and changed over the course of her training. Compared to her medical school self, she had become more adept at emotion work. She acknowledged that there were times in her life when emotion work would be grueling. She would have "bad days" when she'd have to navigate feelings that didn't fit the social situation. But over time, Krista became increasingly emotionally agile – hardly the steady march toward desensitization claimed in the literature. To use her words, she was "wiser and kinder" to herself in fellowship than she was in medical school or even in residency:

> I learned that I have to be kind to myself, but I've also learned that other people will make allowances when you have bad days. And not just make allowances but they will go out their way to be supportive … so all of those things together, learning to have compassion for myself, learning to lean on the people around me, learning how supportive my colleagues were, learning to give myself some time and space – that's been a long journey.

Part of being wiser and kinder was learning to lean on others and give herself some space. And part was learning that feeling rules need not apply:

> I had a moment where I randomly started crying in the middle of the conversation with a resident. I'm like, "I'm so sorry, this has nothing to do with you. I just need a moment." So, not a fun experience but, I think, a valuable check-in with myself.

While crying in front of learners could cause them to wonder, "Is this person capable of being in charge?" it also sends a reassuring message to trainees. No one – not even doctors – are really immune to emotions.

In contrast to the stereotype that medical students are bleeding hearts who care so much and then empathy for their patients declines over time, Krista's story illustrates just the opposite. Having completed residency and fellowship, she had an appreciation for why doctors would compartmentalize feelings. But compartmentalizing and wearing different emotional hats were strategies – they were not ways to care less, but ways to do emotion work. They were not Krista's personal attributes, nor the personal attributes of other doctors in this book. In the course of medical training, Krista's heart wasn't hardened; it became more agile.

CHAPTER FIVE

# Tim's Story About Comfort

since feeling is first
who pays any attention
to the syntax of things
will never wholly kiss you;

wholly to be a fool
while Spring is in the world

my blood approves,
and kisses are a better fate
than wisdom
lady i swear by all flowers. Don't cry
– the best gesture of my brain is less than
your eyelids' flutter which says

we are for each other: then
laugh, leaning back in my arms
for life's not a paragraph

And death i think is no parenthesis
                     – E.E. Cummings, [since feeling is first]

## Introduction: "Feeling is first"

It was one of Tim's rare afternoons outside the hospital when he video-conferenced in from his home office. His medical school, residency, and fellowship diplomas were neatly framed and hanging on the wall behind him. The first months as an attending in a surgical subspecialty had been extremely demanding, with long hours in the operating room. He had expected that. But what struck home for Tim was that he was finally on his own. Just a few months before, when he was a fellow, someone always had his back: "It feels like you're testing the waters, but it doesn't feel like you're totally alone. If something goes badly, you just make a call, and an attending is around in a few minutes." Now there was no one to call. He was the person who was supervising medical trainees. He was the person ultimately responsible for patient care. He was the attending.

Of all the aspiring doctors in this book, Tim was the one with the longest stretch of training: a total of twelve years. "Slow and steady wins the race" could have been Tim's mantra. He had been diligent and purposeful in his pursuit of a career in surgery: medical school, residency, and then fellowship. His diplomas were objective markers of his progress in developing expertise, symbolizing the knowledge he had gained and the skills he had mastered. But it was Tim's subjective sense of feeling comfortable that signaled to him that he was ready to operate unsupervised as an attending. As a resident, he had systematically gained *confidence* in his knowledge and skills. Increasingly, he knew the justifiable "right answer" for almost any surgical problem thrown at him. But confidence could only get you so far, especially when things didn't go according to plan. From Tim's perspective, his *comfort* level was what really mattered.

In the stories these doctors told, confidence slowly grows but is then followed by a deep desire to feel comfortable – the latter being the ultimate signal of readiness for practice and a harbinger of expertise. In distinguishing between confidence and comfort, I take my cue from Tim, who saw confidence as proactive and comfort as reactive:

> I think they're two different terms. I mean, there's a lot of overlap, but I see comfort in a kind of a more – for me at least, when I think about that feeling in the operating room, it's more of a reactive experience. There's an unexpected finding, unexpected bleeding, or some untoward event. It's being able to be comfortable with the unexpected. That's how I conceptualize comfort. Whereas when I think of confidence in the operating room, I think a bit more in active terms. I know the steps in the operation. I'm charting things out actively, prospectively. I think I had confidence before I had what I consider being comfortable in the reactive sense.

In medical school, confidence was at best something students aspired to – a destination far off in the distance – and given the many miles of the marathon still to run, feeling comfortable wasn't even visible on the horizon. Neither confidence nor comfort was discussed with any frequency until after medical school.

The first few years of residency were devoted to building on the knowledge and skills learned in medical school and putting them into practice in a specialty. At this stage in training, doctors in this book talked about the importance of confidence, like how Tim described his "biggest worry" as a resident:

> A metric I am always trying to hold myself against as I am progressing in training is how self-sufficient am I as a surgeon? ... I don't want to be in a position where I feel hesitant to apply certain interventions. I think that is my biggest worry as a resident – that I will undertreat people due to a lack of confidence to do the big-ticket invasive procedures.

Yet there were inklings that feeling comfortable was the finish line for medical training – not confidence, nor competence (the latter the favored verbiage of medical educators). Feeling comfortable was not something trainees could achieve by knowing which treatment to prescribe or technique to employ in which situation. Surgical residents could describe themselves as confident going into the operating room knowing the "textbook" plan for inserting a stent. But as the adage goes, no plan survives first contact with reality.

If a major blood vessel were to unexpectedly tear, surgeons must act immediately to save the patient's life. However, no two tears are alike, and textbook discussions of what to do in such instances are a far cry from repairing one on your own in a patient who has entrusted you with their life. In these situations, confidence was not enough. What mattered was feeling comfortable.

It was when aspiring doctors felt comfortable – and only then – that they declared themselves ready to practice medicine on their own. For example, Alan explained how his level of comfort distinguished his attending self from his resident self:

> As an attending, I have experiences weekly, if not more, that are much more dramatic and much more impactful than the ones I had in residency or in medical school. But the difference is that they don't frighten me. They aren't scary anymore ... I'm more comfortable, less anxious than when I was resident.

For Tim it took four years of medical school, six years of residency, and two years of fellowship to get to the point of feeling comfortable. That signaled to him his readiness to be an attending surgeon:

> I took the right amount of time to get myself to a comfort level in doing what I am doing. That's what I think when I look back on my education and training: I took the time I needed to start this practice in a way that was not going to be unsafe and not going to make me crazy.

## "The syntax of things": Distinguishing comfort from confidence

The study of clinical uncertainty – a phenomenon closely linked to feeling comfortable – dates back to Renee Fox's research in the 1950s.[1] Building on her work, others have studied uncertainty, tolerance for ambiguity, comfort with uncertainty, confidence in clinical decision-making, confidence as a proxy for competence, and more. This body of research tends to focus on how doctors navigate the interconnected complexities of diagnosis and management in clinical practice. In his critical synthesis of this literature, Jon Ilgen and his colleagues defined *certainty* as confidence in one's interpretation of a clinical situation, *comfort* as confidence in one's ability to act safely and effectively, and *comfort with uncertainty* as having the confidence to act on a problem even though one may not be completely confident in one's understanding of the underlying issue.[2] Despite diverse terminology, one thing that research on phenomena related to feeling comfortable has in common is its derivation from cross-sectional research[3] – taking a snapshot of the phenomenon at a point in time. For example, in this kind of research, medical trainees are interviewed and asked to reflect on a particularly perplexing case and how they grappled with making a diagnosis. There's little discussion of how that particular reaction was a product of their past and would contribute to a different reaction in the future. We don't have stories that describe how being confident in one's skills evolves in real time, laying the foundation for feeling comfortable when the unexpected happens because longitudinal qualitative studies are so rare.

In medical education, terms like confidence and comfort are often used interchangeably, and admittedly the distinction between being confident and feeling comfortable is fuzzy. But what I identified in walking alongside six aspiring doctors was a nuanced pattern of when the terms confidence and comfort surfaced over the course of their training. Alan summed up this pattern well one of the last times we spoke. From his perspective as an attending in anesthesia, he recalled his evolution:

> As a medical student and resident, you are constantly uncomfortable. In the back of your mind you're like, "Am I going to hurt somebody? Am I going to do something that is going to be detrimental?" But as you do more and more treatment of patients and more of these dangerous, risky procedures – surgeries, anesthetics – you gain confidence through experience and with that confidence comes comfort in doing the job.

Beyond their sequence was what terms like confidence and feeling comfortable pointed toward. What emerges in the longitudinal data that traces medical trainees from the beginning of medical school all the way into practice is a pattern where confidence was not the ultimate goal; instead, feeling comfortable marked the finish line.

As someone who works in medical education, I was struck that the word competence was so rarely uttered in the interviews. Since the beginning of the twenty-first century, medical education has moved away from relying on time in training as an indirect measure of readiness for practice ("You've completed three years of a rigorous residency, therefore you must be ready") and toward competency-based education as a more direct, objective measure of readiness for practice ("Demonstrate that you have learned the content and then we will know you are ready for practice").[4] But the vernacular of competency-based medical education was not the vernacular of the doctors portrayed in this book. No one declared themselves competent and thus ready for practice as a full-fledged attending physician or surgeon. Nor did any of them say that they were ready for practice when they were told they were ready. In fact, the opposite was often true. For instance, Krista heard from her attendings that she was ready to be on her own, even though she still had two months left in her fellowship. But their words didn't matter; she still felt out of her comfort zone: "I'm between a sense of simultaneously feeling terrified and feeling ready to be my full-fledged professional self."

In this chapter, we showcase Tim's marathon. His story is particularly illuminating for exploring the long trek toward feeling comfortable because responsibilities are granted to surgical trainees incrementally over a long runway: five to seven years for most surgical residencies compared to three years for most medicine residencies (and even then, many surgeons subspecialize and do a fellowship). From Tim, we learn that confidence is a requisite landmark along the way toward feeling comfortable, but it's not the destination. Confidence is a marker of progress – having at one's fingertips a substantial body of knowledge and toolbox of skills. But confidence does not have the same intuitive element as comfort, replacing anxiety with a groundedness that foreshadows expertise. Each of the aspiring doctors in this book was running a different marathon, but what they had in common was knowing that at the end of the race what mattered was feeling comfortable.

## "Will never wholly kiss you": Early days and lacking confidence

Although medicine tends to run in the family (so to speak), none of the trainees in this book had parents who were doctors, making them somewhat of an anomaly.[5] Tim recounted that he wasn't exposed to a career in medicine when he was growing up. He was not premed in college and didn't do much shadowing in hospitals. As a result, Tim mentioned *not* feeling comfortable as first-year medical student:

> I've never quite felt comfortable even with the basic processes that underpin medicine. The simple things, like the timing of the day like when rounds happen or the management of the basic things like lab tests. I feel like I'm playing catch-up in a sense because it's all very unfamiliar.

Tim was not an outlier. The aspiring doctors in this book rarely talked about confidence or feeling comfortable when they were in medical school. In fact, they often spoke of feeling anxious, nervous, or worried. Niki captured the sentiment of many of them when, early in medical school, she explained her anxieties about whether she would be able to rise to the challenge: "I'm so nervous that I might not be able to live up to the standard that I have in my mind for myself or that other people might have in their minds of me as a doctor."

As medical school progressed, Tim and his classmates gained fundamental knowledge about health and disease. They became less reliant on textbooks and more confident in their ability to apply what they had learned. They started to encounter patients with interesting diagnoses such as aspergilloma, a type of fungal infection that can happen after surgery to remove part of a lung compromised by emphysema. Was the routine treatment to cut it out, or to leave it in and manage it medically? It felt like a real accomplishment to Tim and his classmates when they could figure out what the patient needed before being told by someone with more experience. Halfway through his second year of medical school, Tim began to experience the inklings of confidence, even though he admitted he had a long way to go:

> It felt good to have the sense that I could anticipate what was wrong, and I formed an idea with my partner of what could be going on with this patient. Then we looked at his charts, and we were right. Well, we were more often wrong than right, but it was nice to start to think like we were on the right path and be a little more confident.

But the progression toward confidence was hardly an unwavering march forward. The clerkship year of medical school tested the students' burgeoning sense of confidence in what they knew about medicine. They were now officially part of the medical team, and thus the stakes were higher. Alan bluntly described clerkship rotations as a steady stream of moments where confidence was in short supply:

> Clerkships are agonizing because you're constantly feeling uncomfortable and doubting yourself. You don't know what you are doing. It's not even that you don't know what you are doing, but that you could be doing something wrong and not even know it. In the back of your mind, you're like, "Am I going to hurt somebody?"

## "The best gesture of my brain": Residency and the utility of confidence

Despite the lack of confidence that clerkships seemed to induce, all the doctors in this book successfully graduated from medical school and selected a specialty. Tim started medical school thinking he would pursue neurology because it appealed to his baseline interest in philosophy and psychology. However, when he did his neurology clerkship, Tim found the management of chronic neurological conditions to be emotionally taxing and something he preferred to avoid. Conversely, during his surgery clerkship, he discovered that he really liked procedures, so much so that he decided to apply to general surgery residency programs. Tim was accepted into a competitive program that necessitated a major move to a new city and a new academic medical institution.

Consistent with his "slow and steady wins the race" mantra, Tim took the move in stride. What he talked about more than anything else as he transitioned from medical school to residency was the growth of his confidence. As a first-year surgical resident, Tim recalled doing a thoracotomy in the emergency room, "an intense resuscitative thing we do for trauma patients, a last-ditch thing. That's one of the most invasive things we do on an urgent basis." Since confidence was his self-imposed metric of progress, Tim clung to this confidence-boosting experience as a measure of where he stood in training.

> You compare yourself now to where you need to be at the end of training, and it seems like a wide chasm. You hold on to these little moments where you did something important or when you did something critical because they are markers of progress.

Eliza vividly recounted an "amazing moment of gaining confidence" when she was midway through her surgical residency. She was working in the hospital, taking care of patients overnight, when she received a page alerting her to an airway emergency. She recalled telling herself, "I don't want to be the one saving this person's life. It's so freaking terrifying that I just want to let someone else do it." But she was on call and had to face her fears. As things turned out, she successfully secured the patient's airway before the attending arrived and commended her work. In the aftermath, she appreciated the milestone she had reached relative to her confidence:

> I was in a daze and thinking, "Oh my God, what just happened?" It is just a really bizarre moment to be that person getting the airway. And I knew that I needed those three years in residency to feel confident doing that kind of procedure.

As it turned out, confidence was not only an internal indicator of progress but also an external indicator of performance. The doctors in this book talked about acting confident even when they didn't feel confident because they didn't want attendings to take over the clinical task at hand. Any hesitation on their part could be misconstrued as a lack of confidence. To be clear, residents were encouraged to ask for help when they needed it. But they knew that asking for help could signal to a supervising attending that they weren't quite ready to be on their own, and they were loath to miss out on opportunities to learn by doing. Tim put it like this:

> As a surgical learner, you're always balancing a need to learn with a need to display confidence, at least when you're doing something procedural. Sometimes those two things are at odds. If you are voicing uncertainty in a part of a case, maybe that case gets taken from you.

Acting confident wasn't always or even primarily about what residents would gain in terms of their own learning.

Sometimes residents acted confident because they believed that was what patients wanted. As Alan said, residents had to engage patients with confidence so that patients would literally trust them with their lives:

> You need to make them confident that you can do it, make them think like this is something you are going to be able to do relatively easily. It's not going to be a huge stretch for you. You're not concerned about the work you are about to do. Nobody wants their doctor to be concerned.

Projecting confidence also shaped the way aspiring doctors were seen by colleagues. Eliza observed that while giving off an air of confidence may not reflect actual knowledge and skills, it did impact peer opinion: "I'm acutely aware of that and have heard other surgeons say, 'They're not confident, they're not good.'"

Regardless of the rationale, acting confident was not an equal playing field. Women residents had to carefully gauge how they performed or acted confident. On the one hand, they were prone to being written off and doubted if they didn't act confident enough, but on the other hand, acting too confident could land them in trouble. As a male surgeon-in-training, Tim never spoke of having to negotiate his confidence. But as a female surgeon-in-training, Eliza regularly experienced confidence as a double-edged sword:

> It's tough to find a balance between being confident and being too confident. Being a woman and in surgery, you

don't ever want to sound like you don't know what you are doing because people will doubt you – quickly. I can imagine that a lot of women say, "I'll do fine," and take on more than they can handle. There are women who do that and are respected for it. But you can get in deep water. You want to look confident; you want people to know you are competent. So there is that, and then there is turning around and saying, "I don't know what I am doing." You should do that every time [you feel that way], but it's hard because you don't want anyone to think you can't do something.

It's important to note that the doctors portrayed here were quick to distinguish a rising tide of confidence from overweening pride in one's accomplishments. Having too much confidence was problematic. As Niki warned, "You can't ever be too confident and self-assured. You always need to have a little self-doubt. It makes you a better physician because then you will double-check and make sure you are doing everything right for your patients." But for residents, having enough confidence was a psychological safeguard. Tim explained:

> It's not so much pride, although they may come across as prideful. It's more that these moments are kind of psychological stays or buffers. They're experiences that you hold onto because those experiences are relatively few and far between. When you have them, it's important to value them.

## "Life's not a paragraph": The temporality of confidence

All the doctors in this book routinely talked about how their confidence increased during residency, though it was hardly a predictable, straightforward trajectory. For Tim, there were other confidence boosts, much like the thoracotomy in the emergency room, but they were also transient. Confidence was mostly in the rearview mirror, elusive and fleeting:

> When I have these clinical highpoints, when I do something that is lifesaving, independently, I hold on to that because it reminds me that when I am pushed, I can do it. It gives me a little bit of relief against the feeling of dread I have about encountering a clinical scenario where I'm asked to do something, and I'm alone and I can't do it. That is a stress I have all the time. It's not acute, but this lack of confidence lingers in the back of my mind.

For Tim, the ups and downs of residency lasted six years. Surgical residency programs typically set a year or two aside from clinical duties so that residents can design, conduct, and disseminate their research. Like most surgical residents, Tim had gained confidence as his surgical knowledge and skills accumulated over the first two years of residency. But his confidence was challenged in the subsequent two years dedicated to research. Shifting focus from surgical practice to research can be a heavy lift for residents who have limited prior research experience. Tim was not new to research, having done some in college. But doing research in his third and fourth year of residency had higher stakes. As we learned from Eliza, biomedical research was the coin of the realm in research-intensive academic medical institutions like the one where Tim did his residency. Research productivity was valued in this context, and it involved long stretches of time with no definitive markers of progress – and no markers of progress meant no confidence boosts. Tim compared the confidence he experienced in his clinical years to his time doing research:

> In surgery, every day you feel like you really accomplish things. You do three or four surgeries, you have these very discrete tasks, and for the most part, you accomplish them and experience a confidence boost. But research is so different. Things are quite slow-moving. It can be a long stretch between researching something and putting out a manuscript, presenting at a conference, or winning some funding. You wonder: "Am I going to have the chops to do this?"

By the end of his research years, Tim had presented his research internationally and won a national young investigator award. Like the memorable cases previously mentioned, these external validations were confidence boosts that served as markers of progress. And true to form, they did not last:

> I get positive feedback from the people I work with, and I've been awarded for my research. So, to a degree I am on track. But then I look ahead, and I see where I need to be, and

that's always stressful. When I look from that perspective, the confidence dissipates, and it's replaced with the stress of "Am I going to get there?"

Tim shifted his focus back to clinical practice in the last two years of surgical residency. He continued to experience moments of confidence that were a buffer against the creeping anxiety that he wouldn't be ready for practice. With research behind him and clinical work ahead of him, confidence became more familiar and less fleeting. Tellingly, around this same time, trainees seemed more open to asking for help.[6] When they came to understand that being a good doctor was not the same as knowing everything, not knowing something no longer felt daunting. For instance, near the end of his residency, Alan remarked, "The further on you go in training, the more you get confident, and you start making decisions on your own. But you always have to remember that when something comes up that you don't have experience with, then it's totally appropriate to ask someone for help." Asking for help was no longer a sign that residents lacked confidence, as they may have feared earlier in their training.

What had changed? The doctors featured in this book implied that they were starting to lose some of the textbook knowledge they had worked so hard to absorb in medical school. What they were gaining in exchange was a more contextual understanding – a gradual expansion in their zone of comfort. For instance, Blake talked about an increased awareness: "There are situations where the book answer might not be the best answer for the patient and knowing the difference and when to do what." At the end of his residency, Tim explained the phenomenon this way:

> It's kind of reassuring that I'm not relying on abstractions anymore. I've banked enough experience and hours. I'm moving toward, you know, a more intuitive side of practice, which is where you want to be ... I'm realizing that progress through residency is not an absolute metric but maybe instead finding a niche where you're confident *and* comfortable.

## "Kisses are a better fate / than wisdom": The comforts of fellowships

Tim graduated from residency and started a two-year fellowship at the same institution. During his fellowship, he gained increasingly specialized knowledge and skills and secured his place in a surgical subspecialty. While Tim appreciated that the learning curve in fellowship was steep, he wasn't as daunted as he was at the beginning of residency. The confidence he had in his skills had been validated and was now beginning to be buttressed by a subjective feeling of comfort:

> I'm achieving a level of comfort now that I wouldn't have expected during residency, or that at least I didn't experience during residency in the operating room, where I may have been more anxious than others ... this year, as I've finished residency and moved through the first year of fellowship,

there's kind of an internal level of comfort when I'm in the operating room and most things that are happening I'm very comfortable with.

For Blake, feeling comfortable as a fellow was less about technical skills in the operating room and more about practice style. "There is a wide range of acceptable practice, and I'm figuring out where I fall along the spectrum. And figuring what is normal variation that maybe I am not comfortable with, but it is still acceptable." Notably, both Tim and Blake describe feeling comfortable as internal: Unlike confidence, which could be performed, no one talked about "acting" comfortable – they only talked about feeling comfortable. It was as if feeling comfortable entailed *not* having to act. For Tim it meant that even when things went off the rails, he could replace the anxiety he felt earlier with an authentic, calm assurance – a sensation he described as feeling comfortable versus confident: "It's almost like a negative phenomenon. It's like a falling away of that kind of anxiety and just being grounded and comfortable in your practice."

The transition from confidence to feeling comfortable happened for other doctors during later stages of training. For instance, Alan did a four-year residency and then went into private practice. He described the end of his residency as the time when he transcended confidence and used feeling comfortable as the measure of being ready to face challenges:

I don't have anxiety anymore in the operating room. I'm comfortable with almost every situation that comes up.

Things that would have scared me before, like if in the middle of the night, somebody comes in with bleeding that needs to be fixed immediately, right away, or they are not going to make it, are now just "oh, I guess I have to fix that."

Still, there were aspects of fellowships that made this advanced stage of medical training particularly conducive to helping doctors transition from confidence to feeling comfortable. Both residency and fellowship entailed arduous training. But fellows had residency under their belt while still having attendings at hand. According to Tim, this made fellowship a best-case scenario for developing a sense of comfort:

> I don't think a lot of people have that level of comfort at the end of residency, at least in surgery. It's a lot psychologically to go out and get a job with some of these misgivings in the back of your mind. For a lot of people – and myself included, I'll be honest – fellowship is a transition that allows you to kind of inhabit that role but in an environment where you have support readily available and kind of formalized into your experience.

Tim's fellowship ended with what he described as "ideal conditions" for solidifying his feelings of comfort. He was offered a position at the institution where he trained, which meant he experienced a relatively easy transition to being an attending:

> I was in a hospital that I knew really well. I knew just about everyone there. I was doing my own thing. I was operating.

And I even had my own junior fellow who I knew from residency. It was just an amazing way to start ... I was so, so comfortable.

Tim's transition to practice underscores the role of context in affording feelings of comfort. He felt relaxed and secure not only in his abilities but also in his surroundings. He knew the surgical theaters. He knew the wards. He knew the attendings in surgery and in other related fields like radiology. He knew his peers. In his words, "You're comfortable in your own state but also comfortable in your state within your practice environment." Tim not only knew the justifiable "right thing" to do in each scenario that would shield him from the criticism of his peers. He also had reached a stage in his training where he felt comfortable making and defending a different decision if his intuitive knowing pulled him in a different direction.

## Conclusion: "Spring is in the world"

Like the other doctors in this book, Tim expected his knowledge and skills to continue to advance now that he was an attending, but at a slower rate than during residency or fellowship. He would learn something with every case as he fine-tuned his surgical practice. But more important was how he felt comfortable when confronting the unpredictable.

With the borders of his comfort zone expanded, Tim felt prepared to accommodate both improvements in his skill and the unexpected, or as he said, "turbulence in the operating room." He even described the emergence of this state of mind as "kind of like a comfortable onset." Feeling comfortable had truly outpaced confidence, and comfort was his indicator that he was ready to practice as an attending surgeon. And it wasn't until this point that Tim ventured the word "expert." It took twelve years, but at the end of his long arc of training, what mattered was comfort: "I think just being comfortable, that I can be comfortable early in my career and I'm ready to put on the expert hat so to speak."

Indeed, the comfort Tim had acquired extended not just to his surgical practice but even to his conception of himself. He was comfortable in his own skin: "I don't think I'm God's gift to surgery. I think I work hard at it. I'm good at it. I'm safe at it." And most of all, he was comfortable doing surgery safely and effectively:

> One of my favorite quotes from a famous surgeon is, "You don't need to be a Ferrari to do a [fairly complex surgical procedure]. You can be a well-maintained Buick." I think that's true. I don't think I'm a Ferrari of the surgical world. There are only a few of those. I'm happy to be a well-maintained Buick.

Like other doctors in this book who started their medical training at an elite medical school, Tim started out with thoughts of becoming a Ferrari – an award-winning physician scientist. But over the long arc of training, he discovered something unexpected: the flashy allure of being an "all-knowing" Ferrari paled in comparison to being fully functional as a Buick.

CHAPTER 6

# The End of the Arc

> I often passed the Door of Dreams
> But never stepped inside,
> Though sometimes, with surprise, I saw
> The door was open wide.
>
> I might have gone forever by,
> As I had done before,
> But one day, when I passed, I saw
> You standing in the door.
>       – Jessie Belle Rittenhouse, "The Door of Dreams"

## "I saw / the door was open wide": For aspiring doctors, current doctors, and lay readers

The preceding chapters remind us how much we can learn about the transformative process of becoming a doctor by walking alongside aspiring doctors through their training and witnessing their stories. By looking closely at their journeys, we start to grasp how sweeping this transformative process is. Becoming a doctor is not a single transformation. It's not something that you can schedule, much less one you can even anticipate. For doctors-in-training, transformation may not even be easy to explain, as Krista shared:

> I have a hard time articulating exactly how I am different except I know that I am. I was having this conversation with a colleague recently. She graduated with me, and she is now a fellow. Her sister just started an orthopedic residency. Her sister, in a conversation last week, said, "Why didn't you warn me what residency is going to be like?" And the answer is you can't. You just can't comprehend what it is going to be like until you are doing it.

Eliza added that transformation was a slow and subtle process – one that you only recognize toward the end of training: "You get flashbacks every day of what you did, what you had to learn and how much you had to go through to get where you are now. Looking back, you realize you've been transformed." Alan came to medical training with one transformative process behind him (from musician to medical student). In contrast to Eliza's description, his transformation was, as he said, a "whirlwind": "A lot of the stuff in my career is happening in a much shorter time frame than would happen in many other people's careers. I always wonder how much of that is me or how much of that is because I've got this other body of experiences." For Tim, transformation was a maturation, a graceful integration of who he had been, who he was, and who he was becoming. But he and Niki both pushed back on the notion that medical training had transformed them into different people. As Niki put it, "Your personality, and hopefully your morals, and who you are stay the same."

The process of becoming a doctor, whether it's called a transformation, professional identity formation, or constructing a sense of self, is unique for each and every person. And just like the lives that medical trainees live, the process is personalized, dynamic, and nonlinear, making it necessary to study through time. To be sure, there are doctors whose initial conjectures about where they would wind up were spot on. When Tim was a first-year medical student, he said, "Maybe I'll be a surgeon in fifteen years," which turned out to be the case. But even Tim would admit that his journey had its fair share of unexpected twists and turns, peaks, valleys, and plateaus.

A nice, neat package of advice for those on the cusp of the journey to be a doctor would be a fairytale ending. But that is not what the stories of these six doctors offer. Instead, they present paradoxes. In my very last interview, I asked each of them, "What advice would you give to your younger self?" and each responded with a paradoxical insight. For Eliza it was to stay focused on training to be a doctor and yet simultaneously embrace the other things that bring you joy, like music. For Alan it was to do the things that truly interest you, yet not to turn things down if you're not sure you will like them. For Niki it was to hold on to your dreams and at the same time to expect the unexpected. For Krista it was to always have a questioning attitude and still trust yourself to make it work. While Tim and Blake shared similar advice about expecting hard work, they also acknowledged that some of their own success came down to luck – being in the right place at the right time.

Paradoxes help us realize that two things can be true at the same time. But paradoxes don't tell us which truth to pursue. The transformative process of becoming a doctor – starting from medical school and going all the way into clinical practice – isn't about choosing one truth. It's about being able to hold multiple truths at the same time. Medical trainees often are caught in the crosshairs of paradox: How do I hold on to my personal sense of self while at the same time take on the mantle of the medical profession?[1] But trainees almost always complete training, and the doctors in this book eventually figured out how to embrace both. Whether they continue to embrace paradox, I cannot say. That is a project for someone else. What I can say is that my conversations with these aspiring doctors served as a safe space to grapple with paradox – the kinds of things that Eliza said "seem diametrically opposed to each other":

> Our conversations make me think about what I'm doing. I actually wonder how much I have become is because of what you have been doing with me. I don't know if I would have been as introspective about certain things, even though I really love to assess myself. You've asked questions that I've never thought about, things like loving two things that seem diametrically opposed to each other. And that has had to have some effect on me over time.

## "I might have gone forever by": For medical school faculty and scholars in medical education

As I mentioned in the introduction, I wrote this book with various audiences in mind. Hopefully, the stories will resonate with readers who see themselves in medicine and wonder what the future might hold, readers who are doctors in practice and curious about how their story compares to others, and other readers who thirst for doctors' stories, even if they have no plans to enter the medical profession. With my limited use of theory and minimal reference to existing research, I have purposefully not written to satisfy the genre expectations of medical school faculty and scholars in medical education. Indeed, I consistently call out the limitations of tried and true research methodologies, hoping that our field starts to entertain alternatives to relying on snapshots of time or on someone's recollections.

Each of the preceding chapters has argued instead for longitudinal qualitative research to show us how the manifold pasts of these trainees influence their dynamic presents and set the stage for their diverse futures. We need these studies to grasp how powerful social structures of elite medicine shape aspiring doctors far beyond medical school. We need them to understand the agentic choices that medical trainees make in building their careers and how those choices work out for them. We need longitudinal qualitative studies to fully appreciate how trainees in medicine learn not just to avoid burnout at work but to keep life at work in conversation with life outside of work. We need these types of studies to comprehend how doctors learn to manage a range of emotions in the course of their training, including but not limited to empathy. And we need them to notice subtle shifts in how medical students, residents, and fellows talk among themselves about what readiness for practice really feels like.

While the subject matter of the stories told in the chapters is not new to medical education, the length of the stories and how they were positioned through time adds nuanced and often surprising insights to what were often thought of as established verities. Unfortunately, longitudinal qualitative research is notable for its rarity. The lack of this type of inquiry means that there are perspectives about medical training that we may never know, much less be able to use to inform our decisions.

Arthur Frank, a socio-narratologist, writes sagaciously about the use of story in scholarly inquiry. He reminds us that "stories echo other stories," and those echoes bring coherence and meaning to the present story.[2] This struck home to me when, toward the end of the study, I recounted with each of the doctors in this book what they had identified as resonant learning experiences in prior interviews. Although I feared that presenting that information would be a disorienting deluge of data, it was never the case. Instead, each responded like Alan did:

> Each one reads to me like a stepping stone. Each one is, I don't know if it's a requirement for the next one to happen, but certainly each one is a progression. To start off, doing a physical exam on a real patient. By now, I have done hundreds of those and that is not really an interesting thing

anymore. But it was big thing then because it was the first time I was doing it.

Alan talked about these resonant learning experiences as stepping stones – new and often risky experiences that he integrated into his story, tying together his past in ways that dovetailed into his present. He listed them in succession:

- Coming up with a diagnosis and treatment plan for a patient with HIV in one of his clerkship rotations – "The first time my independent thought altered someone's medical treatment."
- Pronouncing someone dead when he was an intern – "Something that only doctors do."
- Performing an emergency intubation under the watchful eye of a supervising attending as a senior resident – "Something that I would never have even dreamed of being able to do as a medical student."

Each stepping stone mattered because it represented an increase in responsibility, an increase in task complexity, an increase in the gravity of what he was doing, and an increase in clarity about who he was as a doctor. Although they may appear disjointed to someone else, they cohered for Alan in a way that made sense to him.

Arthur Frank also writes that stories take on lives of their own, not only as they are retold from person to person but also as they are retold by the same person through time.[3] In recursive interviews in longitudinal qualitative research, participants revise the past and reimagine the future. Often, they remember a critical instance or epiphany but forget the accumulation and configuration of multiple events that preceded it.

The doctors in this book had different reactions when confronting their former selves in recursive interviews. When I talked to Krista near the end of the study, she thought she never had an interest in neonatology until later in medical school. In her personal statement for a neonatology fellowship, she described herself as always intending to pursue a career in obstetrics. According to Krista, it wasn't until she was in her last year of medical school when she had an epiphany in the midst of an emergency C-section and suddenly realized what she really cared about was the baby, not the mother. And yet, eleven years earlier, when she was a rising second-year student coming back to medical school after a summer doing research in pediatrics and shadowing a neonatologist, she told me this:

> I really liked working in pediatrics. I don't think I could be a general pediatrician just doing physicals every day. I think I would get really bored, but working with kids was really great. Whenever I'd go into the hospital with my research adviser, we'd be doing newborn checkups. It was really cool to shadow a neonatologist. So that is something I am seriously considering.

When I pointed out the discrepancy in her stories, Krista replied: "That's the way I have told my story to myself. It has become truth because I've repeated it so often." She told herself and others the story enough times that it became her truth.

To be clear, there is nothing wrong with asking about the remembered past; in fact, sometimes our recollection of critical moments is exactly what needs to be explored. But as psychologist Jerome Bruner reminds us, "Memory and imagination supply and consume each other's wares."[4] The things we can learn by tracing individual journeys to becoming doctors in real time are different from the things we learn by relying on memories of prior phases of training. The aspiring doctors featured in this book remarked on this themselves. For example, Alan spoke to the veracity of what he actually said during our interviews over the years, not what he remembered:

> I could write a memoir, and medical students could read it and get an idea of what my story was. But you have a formal longitudinal study. It's not me remembering, "Oh this was an interesting time," and then writing it down. My memory from twelve years ago is going to be colored, but what you have is concrete – you have a transcript of what I said twelve years ago … And the people who write memoirs – if I write one, it will be subjective and colored by the rose-colored glasses I wear at the time I am writing it. But to have something that is formally collected and the questions you carried through all these years that we can make comparisons to. It's not what I remember saying, it is what I actually said, which is really valuable.

This is not to say that longitudinal qualitative research is immune to critique. Just like any study, it is a product of time and place. It is certainly the case that the data upon which this book is written were generated during seminal medical events that spanned the years 2010 to 2022, from the enactment of Affordable Care Act legislation and genetics-informed personalized medicine to the COVID-19 pandemic and the rise of telemedicine. There were also dramatic social developments during this time, from the legalization of same-sex marriage to the Black Lives Matter and #MeToo movements. These events, to greater and lesser degrees, penetrated the experiences of the doctors featured in these pages. For example, in the middle of the COVID pandemic, Blake struggled to find any sense of balance:

> My professional life is consumed by it, and then I come home and watch the news, and all people want to talk about is COVID. I don't have a zone where I can just talk about life. It's been really hard. I think people in other industries have their work that they can delve into, but for me, going into work is even more in the thick of things.

Another time Eliza related that as a small, Southeast Asian woman, she didn't look like anyone else in her residency program. Instead, her race, stature, and gender made her look like a stereotypical nurse to others – an assumption that she admitted to making herself when interacting with others who looked like she did. She learned to present like a doctor by acting strategically and "being like a guy" – telling dirty jokes and not flinching when hearing them. Acting so may have been disingenuous, but according to Eliza it was also necessary: "Being a woman in surgery, you are just constantly trying to prove yourself, to prove that you are cool and that you are just as normal as guys." Nonetheless, reflections like these were few and far between compared to the overarching themes addressed in the previous chapters. And yet, if the same study were begun today, I would not be surprised if issues like these would move to the fore and others fade into the background. That realization only argues for others in medical education to do more longitudinal qualitative studies.

There is also the unavoidable fact that this book's author is a white female who is a full professor at an institution not unlike the elite, research-intensive, academic institution discussed in Chapter 2. To be sure, the stories in this book were witnessed, curated, and told from my perspective as someone who wants to contribute to medical education. But over the course of my career, I've come to recognize that the same powerful social structures that narrow career choices of medical students also narrow my options for contribution as a researcher. In a *New Yorker* article, writer Adam Gopnik claimed that science is competitive storytelling.[5] In medical education, competitive storytelling is constrained by the coin of the realm: journal articles. But journal articles with 3,000- or 5,000- or 8,000-word limits cannot accommodate stories told over the course of twelve years. Nor do the mandatory structures of introduction, methods, results, and discussion fit well with my penchant for stories. And while it is understandable that as medical education has tried to establish itself as a legitimate field by setting expectations for the use of theory, theory can overshadow story.[6] From where I stand, word limits shouldn't truncate story, structural requirements shouldn't obfuscate story, and theory shouldn't speak louder than the story being told.

## Closing: "I saw you standing in the door"

I want to end by reminding readers that it is the stories of six aspiring doctors in this book that truly matter. I have shared their stories of transformation, but they were the ones standing in the door. To be sure, I listened, asked questions, transcribed, reviewed, and analyzed the qualitative data. In that sense, these stories bear my imprint. But ultimately their stories – not mine – are the teachers.

And while this is the final page of the book, their stories are far from finished. As the poet and essayist David Whyte writes, "*End* is the word that introduces us to an intimacy with, an anticipation of, and even a readiness for new beginnings."[7]

New beginnings aside, one thing has stayed constant: the doctors profiled on these pages are the experts in their own lives. I am forever grateful that they took my invitation to talk as an occasion to reflect on their journey, allowing me to serve as their witness. And to the good fortune of readers, they embraced my invitation as an opportunity to narrate their own growth – a chance to tell their own story.

# A Note to Aspiring Doctors

This book is really for you. While the parts that speak to medical school faculty or scholars may seem too abstract or theoretical, they provide important context and insights into medical education. You can breeze over those parts, but please don't breeze over the stories. Those stories are gifts to you from Blake, Eliza, Alan, Niki, Krista, and Tim. Each one is now a full-fledged doctor. Each one completed the journey through medical training. And each one is continuing to learn what they can about themselves as doctors.

To help you on your journey, the questions below might be useful for reflection or even a small group discussion. They have no right or wrong answers. Consider using them as a starting point for a deeper investigation into your own experiences and aspirations.

## General questions:

1. What was your experience reading this book? In what ways did the book touch you? How did it affect how you feel about becoming a doctor?
2. If you anticipate becoming a doctor, did anything surprise you about what might lie ahead? If you are a medical trainee or a practicing doctor, did the stories reflect any of your own experiences?
3. Whose story were you most drawn to, and why? What aspects of their journey resonated with you the most? What lessons can you take away from their experiences? Conversely, whose story disturbed you? From your perspective, what was it about that story that was troubling?
4. Did reading the book shed light on any potential blind spots that you should be aware of moving forward? Conversely, what part of your story isn't captured in these pages that would be useful for others to know?
5. Each chapter starts with a poem. How might (or how do) the arts provide a useful mirror for your experience as an aspiring or practicing doctor?

## Chapter specific questions:

1. As we discovered in Eliza's story in Chapter 1, elite medical schools are often attractive to aspiring doctors, but they come at a price. For example, elite medical schools tend to value some career options but not others. What

is the culture of medical school you hope to attend/ are attending/did attend, and how has it affected your outlook?
2. Alan's story in Chapter 2 is about agency. Some trainees say they were just lucky to get into medical school or to get into residency. Others say they worked hard to get to where they are. Where do you fall on the "luck" to "hard work" continuum? How do you think this perspective might influence your approach to medical training and your interactions with peers and mentors?
3. In Chapter 3, Niki reached a point where she opted for a job in medicine versus a career in medicine. How do you think about being a doctor – is it a *job*, a *career*, something in between, or something completely different? What factors do you consider essential for being a good doctor and a complete person, and how might they evolve over time?
4. Many people have assumptions about doctors and empathy, specifically that empathy declines in medical training. How did your assumptions about doctors and empathy change after reading Krista's story in Chapter 4? What strategies do you think might be effective in maintaining and cultivating empathy throughout medical training? What other emotions do you believe are crucial for medical doctors to cultivate?
5. Thinking back to Tim's story in Chapter 5, what role do you think the subjective sense of feeling comfortable should play in determining readiness for practice as an attending physician or surgeon? How might these be

balanced with objective measures or further evidence of competence?

Remember, there are no right or wrong answers – only opportunities for deeper reflection and insight. Enjoy the journey, and we'll see you at the end of the long arc of training!

# Notes

**Introduction: Blake's Story About Transformation**

1. Robert Waldinger, "What Makes a Good Life? Lessons from the Longest Study on Happiness," TED Talk, January 25, 2016, video, 12 min., 46 sec., https://youtu.be/8KkKuTCFvzI?si=Ly9Nv7O5NUmT5GxZ.
2. Ingrid Philibert, Betty Chang, Timothy Flynn, Paul Friedmann, Rebecca Minter, Eric Scher, and W.T. Williams, "The 2003 Common Duty Hour Limits: Process, Outcome, and Lessons Learned," *Journal of Graduate Medical Education* 1, no. 2 (December 2009): 334–7, https://doi.org/10.4300/JGME-D-09-00076.1.
3. Ricardo Correa, Maggie Curran, Celeste Eno, et al., "Milestones and Guidebook for Residents and Fellows," ACGME.org, https://www.acgme.org/globalassets/PDFs/Milestones/MilestonesGuidebookforResidentsFellows.pdf.
4. My dissertation work was subsequently published in several papers. See Dorene Balmer, Janet R. Serwint, Sheryl Burt Ruzek, Stephen Ludwig, and Angelo P. Giardino, "Learning Behind the Scenes: Perceptions and Observations of Role Modeling in Pediatric Residents' Continuity Experience," *Ambulatory Pediatrics* 7, no. 2 (2007): 176–81, https://doi.org/10.1016/j.ambp.2006.11.005; Dorene F. Balmer, Janet R. Serwint, Sheryl B. Ruzek, and Angelo P. Giardino, "Understanding Paediatric Resident–Continuity Preceptor Relationships Through the Lens of Apprenticeship Learning," *Medical Education* 42, no. 9 (2008): 923–9,

https://doi.org/10.1111/j.1365-2923.2008.03121.x. Dorene Balmer, Sheryl Ruzek, Stephen Ludwig, and Angelo Giardino, "Pediatric residents and continuity clinic preceptor perceptions of the effects of restricted work hours on their learning relationship," *Ambulatory Pediatrics* 7, no. 5 (2007): 348–53, https://doi.org/10.1016/j.ambp.2006.05.001; Dorene Balmer, Sheryl Ruzek, Stephen Ludwig, and Angelo Giardino, "Learning About Systems-Based Practice in the Informal Curriculum in Pediatric Residents' Continuity Experience," *Ambulatory Pediatrics* 7, no. 3 (2007): 214–19, https://doi.org/10.1016/j.ambp.2007.01.007.

5  This study also resulted in several papers. See Dorene F. Balmer, Christina L. Master, Boyd Richards, and Angelo P. Giardino, "Implicit Versus Explicit Curricula in General Pediatrics Education: Is There a Convergence?" *Pediatrics* 124, no. 2 (2009): e347-e54, https://doi.org/10.1542/peds.2009-0170; Dorene F. Balmer, Christina L. Master, Boyd F. Richards, Janet R. Serwint, and Angelo P. Giardino, "An Ethnographic Study of Attending Rounds in General Paediatrics: Understanding the Ritual," *Medical Education* 44, no. 11 (November 2010): 1105–16, https://doi.org/10.1111/j.1365-2923.2010.03767.x; Dorene F. Balmer, Boyd F. Richards, Angelo P. Giardino, "'Just Be Respectful of the Primary Doc': Teaching Mutual Respect as a Dimension of Teamwork in General Pediatrics," *Academic Pediatrics* 10, no. 6 (2010): 372–5. https://doi.org/10.1016/j.acap.2010.10.001.

6  Longitudinal integrated clerkships (LIC) are a curricular approach to clinical medical education where medical students follow patients along their medical journey, often beginning in primary care and continuing through specialty and sub-specialty care. Medical students are exposed to and engage in multiple medical specialties simultaneously rather than the traditional approach of being immersed in one specialty for a few weeks at a time. A distinct advantage of the LIC approach is that students can foster meaning and enduring relationships with patients and with the doctors who care for those patients.

7  Johnny Saldaña, *Longitudinal Qualitative Research: Analyzing Change Through Time* (Rowman Altamira, 2003).

8  I never suspected when I started this study that I would wind up sharing my research methods in several articles, including why and how to do recursive interviews: see Dorene F. Balmer and Boyd F. Richards, "Longitudinal Qualitative Research in Medical Education," *Perspectives on Medical Education* 6, no. 5 (August 2017): 306–10, https://doi.org/10.1007/s40037-017-0374-9; Dorene F. Balmer, Lara Varpio, Deirdre Bennett, and Pim W. Teunissen, "Longitudinal Qualitative Research in Medical Education: Time to Conceptualise Time," *Medical Education* 55, no. 11 (2021): 1253–60, https://doi.org/10.1111/medu.14542. Nonetheless, I look to

others such as Bren Neale as the real experts; see Bren Neale, *Qualitative Longitudinal Research: Research Methods* (Bloomsbury, 2020).

9  To be clear, each participant routinely agreed to engage in audio-recorded conversation, and I obtained approval from each of the Institutional Review Boards of the institutions I worked at during the course of this study.

## 1. Eliza's Story About Socialization

1  Lauren A. Rivera, *Pedigree: How Elite Students Get Elite Jobs* (Princeton University Press, 2016).

2  W.C. McGaghie, "America's Best Medical Schools: A Renewed Critique of the U.S. News & World Report Rankings," *Academic Medicine* 94, no. 9 (September 2019): 1264–6, https://doi.org/10.1097/ACM.0000000000002742;
Andrew T. Gabrielson and Roy C. Ziegelstein, "Medical School Rankings: Time to End or Time to Amend?," *Academic Medicine* 99, no. 3 (March 2023): 247–50, https://doi.org/10.1097/ACM.0000000000005566.

3  Shamus Khan, "The Sociology of Elites," *Annual Review of Sociology* 38 (2012): 361–77, https://doi.org/10.1146/annurev-soc-071811-145542.

4  An earlier version of my exploration of what medical training in elite medicine accommodates in terms of career interests appears in Dorene F. Balmer, Pim W. Teunissen, Michael J. Devlin, and Boyd F. Richards, "Stability and Change in the Journeys of Medical Trainees: A 9-Year, Longitudinal Qualitative Study," *Academic Medicine* 96, no. 6 (July 2021): 906–12, https://doi.org/10.1097/ACM.0000000000003708. That version did not include information generated when participants were in fellowship or practice.

5  Jeffrey Guhin, Jessica McCrory Calarco, and Cynthia Miller-Idriss, "Whatever Happened to Socialization?," *Annual Review of Sociology* 47 (July 2021): 109–29, https://doi.org/10.1146/annurev-soc-090320-103012.

6  Eliot Freidson, "The Reorganization of the Medical Profession," *Medical Care Review* 42, no. 1 (1985): 11–35, https://doi.org/10.1177/107755878504200103; Frederic W. Hafferty and Donald W. Light, "Professional Dynamics and the Changing Nature of Medical Work," *Journal of Health and Social Behavior* (1995): 132–53, https://doi.org/10.2307/2626961.

7  Tania Jenkins, *Doctor's Orders: The Making of Status Hierarchies in an Elite Profession* (Columbia University Press, 2020).

8  The only comparable study is Jenkins's *Doctor's Orders*. However, her excellent book unpacks status hierarchy in a single medical specialty: internal medicine.

9  "2023 FACTS: Applicants and Matriculants Data," AAMC.org, 2024, https://www.aamc.org/data-reports/students-residents/data/2023

-facts-applicants-and-matriculants-data. These statistics do not include Doctor of Osteopathy schools, which take a whole-person approach to medical practice. Students at DO-granting medical schools go on to practice in all specialties, though such schools traditionally have been "othered" by MD-granting medical schools who have controlled much of the medical profession.

10 James Youngclaus and Julie A. Fresne, *Physician Education Debt and the Cost to Attend Medical School: 2020 Update* (AAMC, 2020).
11 Henry M. Sondheimer, Imam M. Xierali, Geoffrey H. Young, and Marc A. Nivet, "Placement of US Medical School Graduates into Graduate Medical Education, 2005 Through 2015," *JAMA* 314, no. 22 (2015): 2409–10, https://doi.org/10.1001/jama.2015.15702.
12 USMLE Step 1 tests foundational science and its medical applications; USMLE Step 2 tests the application of clinical knowledge to clinical care; and USMLE Step 3 tests medical and biomedical knowledge as well as ability to carry out clinical encounters and tasks in unsupervised medical settings.
13 Jed D. Gonzalo, Anna Chang, Michael Dekhtyar, Stephanie R. Starr, Eric Holmboe, and Daniel R. Wolpaw, "Health Systems Science in Medical Education: Unifying the Components to Catalyze Transformation," *Academic Medicine* 95, no. 9 (2020): 1362–72, https://doi.org/10.1097/ACM.0000000000003400.
14 Rosalyn Maben-Feaster, Maya M. Hammoud, Jeffrey Borkan, Ami DeWaters, Jed D. Gonzalo, and Stephanie R. Starr, *Health Systems Science Education: Development and Implementation*. Vol. 4 of *AMA Meded Innovation Series* (Elsevier Health Sciences, 2022).

## 2. Alan's Story About Agency

1 Mustafa Emirbayer and Ann Mische, "What Is Agency?," *American Journal of Sociology* 103, no. 4 (1998): 964, https://doi.org/10.1086/231294.
2 Emirbayer and Mische, "What Is Agency?," 964.
3 In a recent review, Betancourt and colleagues describe medical students' experience of the minority tax, an expectation that students from underrepresented racial or ethnic backgrounds will assume diversity duties in addition to their academic work. Renée M. Betancourt, Donna Baluchi, Kristina Dortche, Kendall M. Campbell, and José E. Rodríguez, "Minority Tax on Medical Students: A Review of the Literature and Mitigation Recommendations," *Family Medicine* 56, no. 3 (2024): 169, https://doi.org/10.22454/FamMed.2024.268466. Lauren D. Olson provides a much more comprehensive study of inequity in medical schools in her book, *Curricular Injustice: How U.S. Medical Schools Reproduce Inequities* (Columbia University Press, 2024).
4 See https://www.aamc.org/services/member-capacity-building/holistic-review.

5 Dorene F. Balmer, Boyd F. Richards, and Lara Varpio, "How Students Experience and Navigate Transitions in Undergraduate Medical Education: An Application of Bourdieu's Theoretical Model," *Advances in Health Sciences Education* 20, no. 4 (2015): 1073–85, https://doi.org/10.1007/s10459-015-9588-y.
6 This algorithm is intended to minimize bias by standardizing rules and deadlines in the recruitment process. Applicants interview for residency programs they are interested in and are eligible for, and requirements vary by program. Then applicants rank residency programs in order of preference, and programs do likewise. The mathematical algorithm then matches applicants to programs based on these two preference lists, with match results being binding.
7 Karen Evans, "Concepts of Bounded Agency in Education, Work, and the Personal Lives of Young Adults," *International Journal of Psychology* 42, no. 2 (2007): 85–93, https://doi.org/10.1080/00207590600991237.

## 3. Niki's Story About Balance

1 David Whyte, *The Three Marriages: Reimagining Work, Self and Relationship* (Riverhead Books, 2009).
2 Rabia Khan, Brian David Hodges, and Maria Athina Martimianakis, "When I Say... Burnout," *Medical Education* 57, no. 8 (2023): 704–5, https://doi.org/10.1111/medu.15088.
3 "Clinician Burnout: A Crisis in Health Care," National Academy of Medicine, N.d., accessed February 14, 2023, https://nam.edu/wp-content/uploads/2020/08/Clinician-Burnout-Infographic_FINAL_print.pdf.
4 Christina Maslach, Susan E. Jackson, and Michael P. Leiter, "Maslach Burnout Inventory: Third Edition," in *Evaluating Stress: A Book of Resources*, ed. C.P. Zalaquett and R.J. Wood (Scarecrow Press, 1997), 191–218.
5 Rabia Khan, Brian David Hodges, and Maria Athina Martimianakis, "Constructing 'Burnout': A Critical Discourse Analysis of Burnout in Postgraduate Medical Education," *Academic Medicine* 98, no. 11S (2023): S116–S22, https://doi.org/10.1097/ACM.0000000000005358.
6 Ayala Malach Pines, "Teacher Burnout: A Psychodynamic Existential Perspective," *Teachers and Teaching* 8, no. 2 (2002): 121–40, https://doi.org/10.1080/13540600220127331.
7 Pines, "Teacher Burnout," 123.
8 In their scoping review of burnout in post graduate medical education, Khan et al. identify three discourses that represent three ways of conceptualizing burnout. One of these is burnout as existentialism.
9 Schools are a primary entity responsible for the health and development of young people. As such they are an important setting for promoting health and preventing disease, but largely under the purview of school nurses, not pediatricians. See "School Health," AAP.org, February 23, 2022, https://www.aap.org/en/patient-care/school-health/.

## 4. Krista's Story About Emotion

1. Alexandra H. Vinson and Kelly Underman, "Clinical Empathy as Emotional Labor in Medical Work," *Social Science & Medicine* 251 (2020): 112904, https://doi.org/10.1016/j.socscimed.2020.112904; Kelly Underman and Laura E. Hirshfield, "Detached Concern? Emotional Socialization in Twenty-First Century Medical Education," *Social Science & Medicine* 160 (2016): 94–101, https://doi.org/10.1016/j.socscimed.2016.05.027.
2. Arlie Russell Hochschild, "Emotion Work, Feeling Rules, and Social Structure," *American Journal of Sociology* 85, no. 3 (1979): 551–75, http://www.jstor.org/stable/2778583.
3. Sociologists have theorized that clinical empathy has emotional labor. Vinson and Underman argue that consumerism and corporatization in medicine have shaped clinical work such that empathy is routinized performance that helps doctors accomplish what they need to accomplish in clinical spaces. See Vinson and Underman, "Clinical Empathy as Emotional Labor in Medical Work."
4. Hochschild, "Emotion Work," 551.
5. Hochschild rejects an instinctive, more Freudian view where emotions just "flow out," and she rejects Erving Goffman's view that actors simply manage outer impressions. She instead favors an "interactive" account of emotion where social factors don't just prompt emotions but guide them, making emotions "deeply social."
6. Hochschild, "Emotion Work," 563.
7. Mohammadreza Hojat, Salvatore Mangione, Thomas J. Nasca, Mitchell J.M. Cohen, Joseph S. Gonnella, James B. Erdmann, Jon Veloski, and Mike Magee, "The Jefferson Scale of Physician Empathy: Development and Preliminary Psychometric Data," *Educational and Psychological Measurement* 61, no. 2 (2001): 349–65, https://doi.org/10.1177/00131640121971158.
8. Published in 2009, Hojat and colleagues' longitudinal study of 456 medical students who annually completed the Jefferson Scale for Physician Empathy reported a decline in empathy in the third year of medical school. Although other researchers have challenged this oft-cited finding, the trope continues. See Mohammadreza Hojat, Michael J. Vergare, Kaye Maxwell, George Brainard, Steven K. Herrine, Gerald A. Isenberg, Jon Veloski, and Joseph S. Gonnella, "The Devil Is in the Third Year: A Longitudinal Study of Erosion of Empathy in Medical School," *Academic Medicine* 84, no. 9 (2009): 1182–91, https://doi.org/10.1097/ACM.0b013e3181b17e55; Melanie Neumann, Friedrich Edelhäuser, Diethard Tauschel, Martin R. Fischer, Markus Wirtz, Christiane Woopen, Aviad Haramati, and Christian Scheffer, "Empathy Decline and Its Reasons: A Systematic Review of Studies with Medical Students and

Residents," *Academic Medicine* 86, no. 8 (2011): 996–1009, https://doi.org/10.1097/ACM.0b013e318221e615.

9 Some sociologists have pushed back on the "emotion-deficit" understanding of empathy. See Barret Michalec and Frederic W. Hafferty, "Challenging the Clinically-Situated Emotion-Deficient Version of Empathy Within Medicine and Medical Education Research," *Social Theory & Health* 20, no. 3 (2022): 306–24, https://doi.org/10.1057/s41285-021-00174-0.

## 5. Tim's Story About Comfort

1 Renée C. Fox, "Training for Uncertainty," in *The Student-Physician: Introductory Studies in the Sociology of Medical Education*, ed. Robert K. Merton, George G. Reader, and Patricia L. Kendall (Harvard University Press, 1957), 207–42.
2 Jonathan S. Ilgen, Kevin W. Eva, Anique de Bruin, David A. Cook, and Glenn Regehr, "Comfort with Uncertainty: Reframing Our Conceptions of How Clinicians Navigate Complex Clinical Situations," *Advances in Health Sciences Education* 24, no. 4 (2019): 797–809, https://doi.org/10.1007/s10459-018-9859-5.
3 An exception is the work of Georgina Stephens, who has conducted longitudinal qualitative research on how medical students respond to uncertainty, although her work is limited to this one phase of training. See Georgina C. Stephens, Mahbub Sarkar, and Michelle D. Lazarus, "'I Was Uncertain, but I Was Acting on It': A Longitudinal Qualitative Study of Medical Students' Responses to Uncertainty," *Medical Education* 58, no. 7 (2024): 869–79, https://doi.org/10.1111/medu.15269; Georgina C. Stephens, Mahbub Sarkar, and Michelle D. Lazarus, "'A Whole Lot of Uncertainty': A Qualitative Study Exploring Clinical Medical Students' Experiences of Uncertainty Stimuli," *Medical Education* 56, no. 7 (2022): 736–46, https://doi.org/10.1111/medu.14743.
4 The Accreditation Council for Graduate Medical Education (ACGME) began an initiative call the Outcomes Project in 1998 to improve resident physicians' ability to provide safe and effective patient care in complex healthcare delivery systems. The project was intended to shift the focus of residency program requirements and accreditation from process-oriented assessment to an assessment of outcomes in six competency domains.
5 Maria Polyakova, Petra Persson, Katja Hofmann, and Anupam B. Jena, "Does Medicine Run in the Family – Evidence from Three Generations of Physicians in Sweden: Retrospective Observational Study," *BMJ* 371 (2020), https://doi.org/10.1136/bmj.m4453.
6 There is a whole body of literature about discernment or asking for help, separate from but related to the literature on confidence and feeling

comfortable cited earlier in this chapter. See for example Iris Jansen, Renée E. Stalmeijer, Milou Silkens, and Kiki Lombarts, "An Act of Performance: Exploring Residents' Decision-Making Processes to Seek Help," *Medical Education* 55, no. 6 (2021): 758–67, https://doi.org/10.1111/medu.14465.

## 6. The End of the Arc

1 I'd point interested readers to the work of Dr. Adam Sawatsky, in particular his paper about identity and ideology: Adam P. Sawatsky, Caroline L. Matchett, Frederic W. Hafferty, Sayra Cristancho, Jonathan S. Ilgen, William E. Bynum IV, and Lara Varpio. "Professional Identity Struggle and Ideology: A Qualitative Study of Residents' Experiences," *Medical Education* 57, no. 11 (2023): 1092–101, https://doi.org/10.1111/medu.15142.
2 Arthur W. Frank, *Letting Stories Breathe: A Socio-Narratology* (University of Chicago Press, 2012), 37.
3 Frank, *Letting Stories Breathe*, 39.
4 Jerome Bruner, *Making Stories: Law, Literature, Life* (Harvard University Press, 2002), 93.
5 Adam Gopnik, "American Nirvana: Is There a Science to Buddhism," *New Yorker*, July 31, 2017, https://www.newyorker.com/magazine/2017/08/07/what-meditation-can-do-for-us-and-what-it-cant.
6 I write more about the use of theory in this article, Dorene F. Balmer and Boyd F. Richards, "Conducting Qualitative Research Through Time: How Might Theory Be Useful in Longitudinal Qualitative Research?," *Advances in Health Sciences Education* 27, no. 1 (2022): 277–88, https://doi.org/10.1007/s10459-021-10068-5.
7 David Whyte, *Consolations II: The Solace, Nourishment and Underlying Meaning of Everyday Words* (Many Rivers Press, 2025), 100.

# Index

academic medicine, 15–17, 20, 39; and agency, 62, 70–1, 80; and comfort, 146, 151; and emotion, 130–1; and socialization, 41, 48, 54
Accreditation Council for Graduate Medical Education (ACGME), 13–14, 16, 40, 181n4
acute-care medicine, 12, 57, 59, 67, 77, 96, 102
Affordable Care Act, 167
agency, 25, 59–62, 64–6, 71, 75, 80, 162
anesthesiology, 13–14, 20–1, 25, 141; and agency, 59, 68–75, 77–8
anxiety, 139, 143–4, 152–4
arts, the, 56, 58, 63–4, 67, 159–60
attendings, 9, 11, 13–14, 16, 23, 94, 164; and agency, 73–5, 77; and comfort, 136–7, 139, 142, 146–7, 155–7; and emotion, 116, 124, 130, 132; and socialization, 32, 44, 49–50, 52–4

autonomy, 60–1, 75

babies, 93, 121, 125, 132, 165
balance, 25, 83–91, 94–6, 98–9, 101–2, 104–7, 127, 130, 147, 167
bioethics, 43, 131
biomedical research, 13, 24, 76, 84, 131, 151, 178n12; and socialization, 31, 33, 35, 40–3, 49
Bruner, Jerome, 166
burnout, 25, 162, 179n8; and balance, 85–8, 92, 94, 99–100, 106
business administration, 42–6, 49, 53, 78–9

careers, 3–4, 12, 15, 24–8, 161–2, 165, 168; and agency, 57–60, 64–5, 72, 77, 80; and balance, 84–6, 92–4, 98, 104–7; and comfort, 137, 143, 157; and emotion, 109, 114, 122, 130; and socialization, 32–3, 36, 39–40, 44–5

children, 24, 33, 41–2, 51, 69, 102; and balance, 83, 86, 105–6. *See also* babies
chronic diseases, 12, 120, 145
clerkships, 11–12, 18–21, 164, 176n6; and agency, 67–8; and balance, 91, 93; and comfort, 144–5; and emotion, 115–16, 120–1, 129; and socialization, 40, 44
clinical medicine, 2, 10–13, 15–17, 161, 176n6; and agency, 56, 63, 68, 70, 74, 77–80; and balance, 86–7, 100–1, 103; and comfort, 140, 147, 150–2; and emotion, 109, 115–17, 130–1; and socialization, 35–6
colleagues, 77–8, 84, 97, 101, 159; and comfort, 148, 156; and emotion, 120, 125, 133
college, 10, 15, 30–1, 38, 63, 90–2, 115–16, 130, 143, 151. *See also* universities
comfort, 26, 77, 101, 137–43, 152–7, 182n6; and emotion, 125–6
community hospitals, 130
compartmentalization, 110–11, 127–8, 134
compassion, 109, 113, 128, 133
competence, 14, 26, 40, 138, 140–2, 149, 154, 174, 181n4
competition, 10–11, 62, 131, 145, 168; and socialization, 36, 38–40, 48
confidence, 3, 8, 26, 73, 93, 181n6; and comfort, 137–55, 157
COVID-19 pandemic, 87, 103, 131, 167
cross-sectional studies, 4–5, 140
curricula, 11, 17–18, 34, 176n6

death, 74, 84, 97, 103, 110, 125, 136; and emotion, 114, 126

decision-making, 75–6, 103; and careers, 23, 26–7, 33, 43, 46–7, 59–65, 72, 92, 105; and comfort, 140, 152, 156, 163
diagnoses, 14, 128, 140, 144, 164, 6161
discoveries, 35, 38, 41, 76
diversity, 27, 63–5, 178n3

efficiency, 11, 42, 96
electives, 12, 42, 45, 56, 68, 102
elite medical schools, 24, 84, 122, 157, 162, 172, 177n4; and agency, 58–9, 62, 65, 67, 70–1, 76, 80; and socialization, 30–45, 51–4. *See also* faculty, medical school
emergency medicine, 13, 47, 84, 164; and agency, 56, 67, 74; and comfort, 146, 150; and emotion, 120, 125
Emirbayer, Mustafa, 59–61
emotions, 26, 108–14, 116–17, 119–34, 163, 180n3, 180n5, 181n9; and comfort, 137, 142–5, 153–6
empathy, 26, 111–14, 117–19, 121–3, 132, 134, 163, 180n3, 180n8, 181n9
employment, 2, 10, 19, 31–2, 141, 155, 173; and agency, 64, 68, 73, 78–80; and balance, 83–4, 87, 92, 95, 98, 100–5; and emotion, 112, 123, 130; and socialization, 41, 43–4, 48, 53
ethnography, 17–19
exams, 3, 12, 14, 36
exhaustion, 85, 88, 92, 96–7
expertise, 137, 143, 157, 169, 177n8
extracurricular activities, 10, 42, 56, 65, 97

faculty, medical school, 28, 62, 68, 94, 118, 162, 171
failure, 122
families, 21, 25–6, 69, 77, 143; and balance, 83–4, 90, 97, 99–102, 104–7; and emotion, 115, 117, 119–20, 125–6, 132. *See also* children; marriage; parents
feeling rules, 113–14, 124–5, 133
fellowships, 10–11, 13–15, 21, 26, 100, 159, 163, 165; and agency, 71, 76; and comfort, 136–7, 139, 142, 153–6; and emotion, 129–34; and socialization, 30, 32–3, 35, 39, 43, 50–4
Fox, Renee, 140
Frank, Arthur, 163–4
frontline providers, 26, 129–30
funding, 24, 31–3, 54, 151
futures, 2, 5–6, 12, 32, 38–9, 140, 162, 164; and agency, 60–3, 66–7, 70, 80; and balance, 82, 104

gap years, 30, 44, 53
gender, 167–8. *See also* men; women
general medicine, 12–15, 21, 75–6, 145, 165
goals, 26; and agency, 58, 66; and balance, 84, 86, 92–4, 98, 100, 106; and socialization, 33, 37, 41–3, 47, 51, 54
growth, 7, 22, 63, 146, 169
gynecology. *See* obstetrics and gynecology (OB-GYN)

Harvard Study of Adult Development, 6
healthcare resources, 14, 42, 45, 54, 100, 104
health systems science, 14, 18, 24, 33, 87, 100; and socialization, 35, 40–2, 45–50, 53

HIV/AIDS, 57, 164
Hochschild, Arlie, 112–13, 180n5
hospitals, 2, 8, 12, 15–16, 18, 20, 165; and agency, 57, 74, 77; and balance, 94–6, 98–100, 103–4; and comfort, 136, 143, 146, 155; and emotion, 116, 120–3, 130; and socialization, 36, 50, 53–4. *See also* children's hospitals

identities, 3–4, 20, 34, 100, 160, 182n1; and emotion, 109, 124
Ilgen, John, 140
illnesses, 56–7, 87, 97, 117
immigrants, 100–1
initiative, 65–6
inpatient medicine, 12, 18, 63, 102
intensity, 10, 12–13, 27, 96, 103, 142, 146; and emotion, 111–12, 116, 118, 120, 122–3, 127–9, 131
intensive care units (ICUs), 96, 130
internal medicine, 11, 13, 45, 68
international medicine, 41–2, 177n8
internships. *See* residencies
interviews, 18–20, 22–3, 28, 160, 163–6, 176n8; and comfort, 140, 142; and socialization, 30, 39
interviews, medical school, 10, 12, 36, 179n6

Jefferson Scale of Physician Empathy, 114
jobs. *See* employment

Khan, Shamus, 33
knowledge, 14, 26; and agency, 71, 73, 76–7; and balance, 90, 99; and comfort, 137–8, 141, 143–5, 148, 150, 152–3, 156; and socialization, 35, 38, 40

leadership, 35–6, 38, 75, 79, 94, 134
life-changing situations, 2, 56–7, 59–60, 77
lifestyles, 12, 59, 68–9, 83, 85–6, 89, 98–9. *See also* balance
loans, 12, 37, 69
longitudinal studies, 5–8, 15, 21–2, 28, 34, 61, 162–8, 180n8; and comfort, 141, 181n3

marriage, 21, 61, 69, 83–5, 99–102, 130, 167
Maslach Burnout Inventory, 87, 89
meaning, 25, 33, 58, 67, 127, 163, 176n6; and balance, 88–9, 93, 97, 104–6
Medical College Admissions Test (MCAT), 11, 36, 64
medical education, 3–9, 15–18, 21, 24–8, 60, 162–3, 168, 171, 176n6, 179n8; and balance, 85, 88; and comfort, 138, 141–2; and emotion, 111, 114, 118, 130; and socialization, 34, 40–1
medical practice, 23, 27, 162–3, 178n9; and agency, 68, 77; and comfort, 139, 152, 154; and socialization, 35, 46
medical school, 2–3, 7–13, 18–23, 25, 27–8, 161–2, 165, 171, 178n9; and agency, 58, 62–8, 75, 80; and balance, 84, 90–3, 95–6, 98, 103, 105–6; and comfort, 136–9, 141, 143–5, 152; and emotion, 112, 115–16, 119, 121–4, 130, 133; and socialization, 30–8, 40–2, 45, 49, 53. *See also* elite medical schools; faculty, medical school; medical training
medical school applications, 10, 36, 62–3, 65. *See also* interviews, medical school

medical students, 2–4, 8, 10–13, 18–22, 95, 159–60, 163–8, 176n6, 178n3, 180n8; and agency, 60, 62, 65–6, 72, 76–7; and balance, 84, 89–90, 94; and comfort, 138, 141, 143, 181n3; and emotion, 111, 114, 116–19, 123–4, 134; and socialization, 32, 35–7, 39, 41–3. *See also* elite medical schools; medical school; medical training
medical training, 2–7, 9–10, 12, 16, 21, 24, 27–8, 158–63, 166, 171; and agency, 60–1, 68–9, 75, 77–8; and balance, 85–8, 94, 97, 99; and comfort, 136, 138–43, 146, 152, 155–7, 181n3; and emotion, 109, 111, 114, 118–19, 124, 127, 129–30, 133–4; and socialization, 35, 39, 41, 43–4, 50. *See also* elite medical schools; medical school; medical students
memories, 5–6, 11, 151, 166
men, 62, 148
mental health, 86, 90, 97, 100–2. *See also* exhaustion
mentors, 52, 99–100
minoritization, 62, 178n3
Mische, Ann, 59–61

National Residency Matching Program, 70
neonatology, 26, 130–1, 165
neurology, 11, 145
Nobel Prize, 41
nurses, 120, 130, 167, 179n9

obstetrics and gynecology (OB-GYN), 11, 25, 91–5, 106, 165
occupational health, 103
on call, being, 2, 56, 69, 146
oncology, 12, 84, 97

operating rooms (ORs), 45, 59, 72–4, 79; and comfort, 136–8, 153–4, 157
orthopedic surgery, 12, 159
outpatient medicine, 63, 72, 102

pain, 97, 108–10, 120; and agency, 57, 71, 74, 78
parents, 84, 86, 103, 114, 128, 132, 143
patient care, 2, 8, 11–14, 16, 26, 176n6; and agency, 56–8, 68, 71, 73–5, 78; and balance, 95–7, 100–1, 103, 105; and comfort, 136, 139, 141, 144, 146, 148–9, 152, 181n4; and emotion, 109–11, 114–20, 122–9, 132; and socialization, 31, 40–2, 44–5, 50
pediatrics, 2, 11–14, 17–21, 25–6, 130, 165; and agency, 75–6; and balance, 83, 93–5, 100–3, 106. *See also* babies
personal lives, 83–6, 89, 96–8, 112, 161–2, 169; and balance, 99, 101–2, 104, 107
personal protective equipment (PPE), 131–2
physical exams, 8, 116–17, 163, 165
Pines, Ayala, 88
pregnancy, 102–4, 120–1, 132
prerequisites, 10, 64, 71, 115
prestige, 33–4, 39–40, 51–2, 59, 80, 83. *See also* elite medical schools
primary care, 11, 25, 68, 176n6; and balance, 100–3, 106
private practice, 25, 71, 77–9, 130, 154
privilege, 34, 77, 168
procedures, 14, 21, 46, 91–2, 138, 141, 145, 147, 157; and agency, 56, 59, 64, 68, 72, 78
psychiatry, 6, 11–12

psychology, 67, 88, 128, 145, 149, 166
public health, 42–3, 103
pure medicine, 24–5, 41

qualitative research, 17–18, 20–2, 28, 34, 141, 162–9, 181n3

race, 167, 178n3
recognition, 31, 48, 53, 57. *See also* elite medical schools
relationships, 18–19, 52, 176n6; and balance, 85, 98–9, 103; and emotion, 115–17, 120, 129
reproductive health, 106
research, 10, 12–13, 15, 17, 86, 162, 165, 168; and agency, 70–1; and comfort, 140, 150–2; and emotion, 114, 131; and socialization, 31, 33, 35, 40, 44, 54. *See also* biomedical research
residencies, 2, 6–14, 17, 19–23, 25–6, 159, 163–4, 167, 179n6; and agency, 60, 66, 68–78; and balance, 94–100, 102, 106; and comfort, 136–9, 141–2, 145–53, 155–6, 181n4; and emotion, 110, 112, 122–7, 129, 131, 133–4; and socialization, 31–2, 35, 38–40, 43–4, 46–53
responsibility, 2, 8, 13, 53, 68, 74, 95, 105, 164; and comfort, 136, 142; and emotion, 123–4
rotations, 11–13, 16, 145, 164; and agency, 68, 73–4; and balance, 93, 97, 102; and emotion, 115, 128–9; and socialization, 44–5
rounds, 2, 14, 20, 75, 143

salaries, 12–13
scholarships, 32, 37
school-based health, 102–6, 179n9
scutwork, 71–2, 78
self-care, 86, 113

senior residents, 13–14, 73, 75
shadowing, 36, 102, 143, 165
shifts, 2, 13, 47, 56, 83–4. *See also* work hours
skills, 8, 12, 14, 18, 21, 26, 45, 48, 101; and agency, 56, 64, 71, 77–9; and comfort, 137–8, 141, 143, 148, 150, 153–4, 156; and emotion, 117, 131
socialization, 21, 32–6, 39–40, 60, 112–14, 162
social relations, 17, 24–5, 100–2, 117, 121, 125–6, 133, 162, 167–8, 180n5
specializations, 10–12, 14, 18, 21; and agency, 58, 60, 67–72; and balance, 91–2, 98; and comfort, 138, 145, 153; and emotion, 115, 124; and socialization, 33, 35, 44–6, 49, 52. *See also* subspecializations
staffing, 79–80, 94
status hierarchies, 34–5, 60, 66, 177n8
stress, 25, 38, 112, 119, 127, 150, 152; and balance, 84–6, 95, 106
studying, 10, 30, 36, 89–91, 131
subspecializations, 12, 14, 68–9, 176n6; and comfort, 136, 142, 153; and emotion, 130; and socialization, 30, 39, 48, 51
success, 1, 85, 87, 90, 125, 156, 161; and socialization, 31–2, 37, 40, 44, 52, 54
supervision, 8, 13, 16, 53, 164, 178n12; and agency, 68, 73–5, 78; and comfort, 136–7, 147
surgery, 2, 9, 11–12, 14, 20, 23–4, 26, 160, 167; and agency, 57, 59, 65, 67–9, 71–3, 76–7; and balance, 91–2, 94, 98–9, 106; and comfort, 136–9, 141–2, 144–8, 150–3, 155–7; and emotion, 126–9; and socialization, 30, 33, 39, 41, 43–53

teaching, 11–13, 33, 52, 63, 75, 169; and emotion, 114, 118–20
television, 4, 27, 47
temporality, 59–61, 64, 70, 88, 160, 166
transformative processes, 2–5, 7–9, 21, 23, 27–8, 158–61
tuition, 13, 32, 37

uncertainty, 38, 46, 140, 156, 160, 181n3
underserved populations, 24, 33, 41–2, 45, 47, 51, 53, 100–1
United States Medical Licensing Examinations (USMLE), 12, 40, 178n12
universities, 15–16, 31, 84. *See also* college

vacation, 3, 104
values, 31, 58–9, 62, 71, 80, 149
volunteering, 10, 36

well-being, 86, 90, 99, 111, 123
White, David, 83–4, 169
whiteness, 62, 168
women, 52, 148–9, 167–8
women's health, 114
work hours, 2, 13, 44–5, 136, 161; and agency, 55–6, 69, 80; and balance, 84, 95–9, 101, 104; and socialization, 48–9
workplaces, 25, 88–9, 104, 123, 156

www.ingramcontent.com/pod-product-compliance
Ingram Content Group UK Ltd.
Pitfield, Milton Keynes, MK11 3LW, UK
UKHW011241091225
465720UK00010B/169